The Pace Of Grace

A NEW ENERGY FOR A CHANGING WORLD

By Karina Joy Stephens

Karina Joy Stephens C/- Intertype
Unit 45, 125 Highbury Road
BURWOOD VIC 3125
www.intertype.com.au

Ordering Information:
Quantity sales. Special discounts are available on quantity purchases by corporations, associations, and others. For details, contact the "Special Sales Department" at the address above.

The Pace Of Grace/ Karina Joy Stephens. —1st ed.
ISBN 978-0-6450010-4-4

Contents

Dedicated to the most generous man I know: my husband, Ian, who supported me unconditionally on my sabbatical of wellness; and for my fur babies, Diggity and Delhi, who sat by my side the whole time I was writing and kept me company. And to all the guests who graced our doors at enRich Retreat & Spa, may you forever life at the Pace of Grace.

NOTE TO READERS

This book was originally titled "The StressLess Revolution – How to live your Best life without getting burnt out, stressed out, maxed out and checked out". It was first printed in 2015.

In October 2020, I decided to update the book and rename it. My decision to do so was based on the events of 2020 and a deep knowing that the content of this book was meant for such a time as this.

Who would have thought that the world would have changed the way it has and that we would be living life with so much uncertainty? As I stood back and observed how people have adapted, I saw so much fear and stress in so many lives including my own.

The world has changed and in order for us to evolve we need to change with it. There is a new energy on earth. The way we have done things in the past needs to change in accordance with this new energy. It is now easier to tap into flow and move out of stress and struggle. The way we do this is to change our energy and this book will help you to do just that.

My prayer is that you find peace in the uncertainty, calm in the chaos, and joy in the unknowing.

This publication contains the opinions and ideas of its author. It is intended to provide helpful and informative material in the subject addressed. The strategies outlined in this book may not be suitable for every individual, and are not guaranteed or warranted to produce any particular results.

There is also the use of minor cussing which I have opted to leave in because it describes perfectly the way I was feeling at the time, so if this bothers you I apologise, it is not meant to offend in any way.

This book is sold with the understanding that neither the author nor the publisher is engaged in rendering medical, psychological, nutritional, or other professional advice or services. The reader should consult a competent professional before adopting any of the suggestions in this book or drawing inferences from it.

No warranty is made with respect to the accuracy or completeness of the information or references contained herein, and both the authors and the publisher specifically disclaim any responsibility for any liability, loss or risk, personal or otherwise, which is incurred as a consequence, directly or indirectly, of the use and application of any of the contents of this book.

What's your energetic signature?

Change your energetic signature,
transform your life?

Interested?

Take the free masterclass and learn how to analyse your energetic signature and then learn how to change it in order to transform any area of your life.

Visit the link for more info

https://www.karinastephens.com/ayes-landing/

Introduction

What is the Pace of Grace?

We say enough's enough to the fast-food, fast-paced, ASAP rat race we call life, and we pause long enough to see what it is doing to us.

Then we consciously lean into some lifestyle changes, which will make us more beautiful inside and out. That will replenish every cell in our body and eliminate disease, illness, and sickness. That will build our resilience so that we can bounce back from life's knocks a whole lot quicker and easier. Stress levels will reduce, and inflammation and toxicity in the body will begin to recede.

These changes will also allow life to begin to flow with effortless ease and grace, just like it is supposed to, as we begin to take our hands off the wheel and trust in the divine process.

It's a way of life, which nurtures and supports the mind, body, and spirit. It's about stripping back all the toxic stuff, which is literally killing us and making us less than what we should be.

Here we take the time to stop and marvel at life. We breathe and exhale, and really learn what it feels like to be totally present with ourselves.

Then we begin to give a little love back to our self by being kinder and gentler. We nourish rather than deplete, and enrich our lives with the kind of things that make our bodies and our souls squeal with delight.

It's not about doing more, having more, and wanting more. It's about doing it differently: appreciating the things you do have and wanting the things that make you feel good naturally. All the while, still having your big dreams and goals, and desiring the good things in life. It's funny, but as you slow down, these things come to you faster and more organically. It's definitely a much nicer place to manifest from, trust me.

It's time to give back to yourself; it's time to feel so tingly alive it's scary. It's time to have the energy, passion, and exuberance you were designed to have. Most of all, it's time to love yourself and this amazing planet we call home.

Struggle depletes us; challenges energise us. You don't have to struggle to know affluence and joy; it's about being in a higher vibration.

You now hear the still, small whisper; your intuition is stronger. You pay attention. Your vibration is higher; you attract circumstances and situations which benefit you and your dreams.

You have energy; your body is alive. Your cells are tingling. Desires seem to appear faster, but still in the Pace of Grace. This pace is slower; it's calmer and effortless. There is a subtle energetic movement, which carries you along. It is not free of crisis, yet as you journey along you become more resilient, stronger, healthier, and wiser.

Things don't affect you like they used to. You have changed certain beliefs; you have had a physical shift and a cellular change. Your nervous system has repaired itself. You have made friends with stress. You have found the courage to look at your feelings and inquire after them. They talk to you and tell you what is wrong; they rejoice in your awareness.

If you are looking for a Band-Aid approach for dealing with stress then this book is not for you. If you aren't prepared to get a little uncomfortable in order to overcome stress, struggle, and fatigue forever, then I suggest you put this book down now. The Pace of Grace is about going deep in order to get permanent results.

In 2012, I was stressed out, burnt out, maxed out, and checked out. I was a girl who had a desire to make a difference with her life and now I had run out of oomph.

This book is about how I was able to let go of the struggle, stress, and burnout, and begin to live a life of ease, joy, and abundance. Stress was literally blocking my life force in all areas and once I realised what the blocks were, I could identify how to release them from my life.

I share how I physically restored my body back to its natural state, thereby reducing years of built-up toxicity, calcification, cellular atrophy, and just plain worn-out organs and systems. In the process, I created a stress defence shield where stress could no longer affect me like before.

I also looked at what was causing stress in my body emotionally and how I shifted old self-sabotaging beliefs which were no longer serving me. I show you how you can burst through any limiting belief in minutes.

By addressing my energy system I was able to remove energetic blocks, which I had no idea were completely deflecting any chance of ease or abundance into my life. The Pace of Grace contains the meditations, guided visualisation, and energy medicine techniques which I used to do this.

Then I looked at what I needed to do spiritually in order to align myself up with my divine purpose, receive direct guidance from Source, and completely transform my life. This book is a journey on how to access your divine potential and release your soul's highest expression.

What I found was a rhythm and a beat to life, which was so different than the one I had been dancing to before. This one was softer, slower, and gentler.

The slower I went, the deeper I got, and the faster I seemed to get to where I needed to be. I realised I was accessing what I have come to term the Pace of Grace. Grace not from a religious definition but to me it means peace, joy, abundance, surrender, and love. Free from anxiety, striving, and struggle.

The only way to access the Pace of Grace is through slowing down. It's not about giving up on your dreams and living off the grid. It's about doing life without all the white noise and static. We're dialled into the wrong frequency and we need to find the one that breathes life into our souls.

It's living authentically and getting on with your mission in the world without the struggle and the push, push energy. You are starting a StressLess Revolution in your own backyard.

I think of it as revolution through evolution. It's about creating a new way by first evolving our self. It is not about forcing change, as this serves no one. We need to dissolve the hardness of years of conditioning with the softness of a new skin.

This is a holistic approach to living a StressLess life. We cover the physical, emotional, the mindset, and the spiritual. Even if you only adopt one or two principles from this book your life will be changed.

The Pace of Grace offers you the tools and inspiration to begin to experience revolutionary transformation.

It is my prayer that you be inspired to start thinking of new ways of living. By adopting a StressLess diet you begin to heighten your intuition. By slowing down physically, you tap into a life force that is free of striving.

The book encourages you to get off the rat race of life and lean into some lifestyle changes that will provide abundant energy, enhanced instinct, and intuition, which will guide you to your divine purpose in life quicker.

This means that we are going to need more energy, more stamina, more passion, more drive and if you have just read this sentence and are thinking, *Struth, I can't even make it through a normal day and this chick is telling me I need to do more*, hold on a sec before you throw this book across the room.

You can have more of everything I mentioned by doing less physically and more energetically. Yes, you read right. You can live life full out, chock-full of vitality and energy. You can live your dreams, create the life you want all without the stress, struggle, and fatigue most of us are experiencing in our lives today.

When you remove the blocks that stress causes, life moves closer to you. It's not about you chasing anything; it's about removing what is stopping life coming to you.

Now, before we move forward, I want to address some of the wording in this book so that it doesn't become a block for you. I do use the word God and if this does not resonate with you then please just insert your own word. I write it because this is how I talk and if I was to change this in order to please the masses I would not be acting authentically.

This is a personal development book with a spiritual bent, and a health and wellness component thrown in to round it off. We cannot live fully if we do not have these areas of our lives working, and as this is a book about being the best person you can be, we need to cover off on all these areas. If you are new to personal development or spirituality, some of the healings, meditations, and visualisations may seem a bit strange to you; this is okay. We all find our own original medicine which heals and reveals so if you are not resonating with anything, just don't add that particular tool to your cute little tool belt. It will always be there if at some point down the track you think to yourself, *You know what, I think I believe in angels now.*

As I have mentioned, this was my path to overcoming a situation which completely debilitated me. I am no different than you, except that I have a different story to share. It is our stories which connect us, which transform lives and bring hope to hopelessness. That is why I share my stories. I am not an avid researcher; I am not a scholar; I don't overly relate to statistics or cold, hard facts. I live life by feeling into it, I make choices based on my idea of common sense, and I am guided by my intuition on every decision I make. If something needs to be proven, I don't always have to have science to back it up; most of the time, actual life experience is proof enough.

I have seen first-hand how stress, struggle, and fatigue can knock you out of the game of life, to the point where you resemble nothing of your glorious self. I was the one who championed the underdog because I was the underdog. I was the girl with the big dreams of changing the world. I was the one attending all the seminars and conferences around the world just so I could live my dream. I was the person in the self-help section of the bookshop buying every book I could and I was the one who would struggle and never, ever give up.

And then life threw me a curve ball and taught me that there is a different way. One where I could have everything I wanted and more, only without the stress. Through my healing came my revealing and with that revealing, a vision of an idea whose time has come. An idea where if we could remove the blocks to our highest self, caused by stress, then we could ultimately awaken to a more peaceful existence. If we changed the stressful thoughts we could ultimately change the direction of the planet. And if we stopped causing the stress on our beautiful animals and this amazing planet we would create a world where kindness is our legacy.

So sit back, relax, allow a deep breath, and allow grace to wash all over your beautiful, magnificent body.

Karina Joy Stephens xxoo

CHAPTER 1

Accessing Grace

"There is a way of living in the world that is not here although it seems to be. You do not change your appearance although you smile more frequently, your forehead is serene and your eyes are quiet."
A Course in Miracles

They said that the twenty-first of December 2012 was a significant date in history: the closing of a chapter, a window of possibility for an evolutionary leap. Looking back now, I happen to believe that the twenty-first of December was the end of my life as I knew it, for a couple of reasons. The first was because I was about to embark on one of the most soul-transforming journeys of my life. The second was because that was the day my husband's extended family, totalling twelve, all came to my house for a Christmas holiday, which was to last ten days. Now, I totally love these guys, but I went into meltdown, I was stressing about everything. Some would say there is nothing wrong with that; it's perfectly understandable, but it was more of a "holy shit" moment than it should have been. It was actually the straw that broke the camel's back.

After Christmas, I started to have major exhaustion episodes. I would need to lie down in the middle of the day and would sleep for hours. Even if I slept for ten hours at night, I would still wake up exhausted.

I would sit in front of my computer and experience a severe sense of overwhelm. I literally couldn't do anything. I could not exercise without being fatigued for the rest of the day. I had run out of juice; there was no excitement or inspiration for me anymore. This was so not me!

I didn't handle stressful situations like I used to anymore; my response now was to go into meltdown. Normally I would tell myself to suck it up and move on. Now I was reacting like I had never-ending PMS. Permanently checked out is what I was.

Within the space of a month, my father was diagnosed with cancer, my father-in-law suffered heart failure and nearly died, and my spa manager resigned. And the hits just kept on coming.

I believe wholeheartedly in natural medicine, so I took myself off to an Integrative General Practitioner and asked for a hormone-saliva test. I thought I may have been going through menopause; it was either that or cancer, I surmised, with just a dash of drama-queen diagnosis.

The week I was scheduled to get the results was probably one of the most challenging weeks of my life. I was driving back from a trip to the supermarket with my husband, Ian. All of a sudden, he pulled off the road and into a little secluded park. My first response was that he wanted to go parking in the middle of the day, and I remember thinking, *Cheeky bugger, it's broad daylight. This will be interesting.* A midday romp was not on the cards, though, as my husband proceeded to inform me that we were going to lose one of our companies due to bad financial advice, and we could be liable for hundreds of thousands of dollars in repayments. Talk about being sideswiped; I was completely stunned.

Call it a sign of things to come, but as we drove home, it started to rain. When we reached our driveway, the wind had picked up so much that debris was being blown in all directions. We scrambled indoors, and within a matter of minutes, the power went out; what followed was a mini hurricane that lasted all night. We were trapped inside with nowhere to go. I couldn't run from my problems; I had to face them head on.

The next day, we were cleaning up the aftermath when the doctor called me in for the results of my tests. I was diagnosed with stage-two adrenal fatigue. She advised me to take a number of supplements, rethink my lifestyle, and reduce stress in my life. F*%k!

I went home and Googled everything I could: What is adrenal fatigue? How did I get it? What is the cure? What are the effects? I was like a dog with a bone. In my research, I looked at not only the physical cause but the emotional one as well. Being a licensed teacher in Louise Hay's *Heal Your Life* work taught me that without looking at the emotional system, you can never fully get to the root of the cause.

What I learned was that about 80 percent of people now have some form of adrenal burnout. And what this basically means is that we are just plain tired. A major "aha" for me was when I realised that I was so tired of the struggle and strain of life, of always feeling like I had to fight to make things work, to get ahead. I had lived this way my whole life, and now my body was saying something had to change.

I was determined to regain my wellness, and after a week, I had come up with my game plan. My research told me that if I do everything right, it will take six to twelve months to fully recover my energy levels. I was going to step down as managing director of my spa and become managing director of my well-being. I gathered a support team, informed them of my needs, and went to work on healing myself. I was taking a sabbatical into wellness.

Through addressing my nutrition, my beliefs, and my lifestyle, I accessed a rhythm and flow to life, which turned my whole way of seeing the world upside down. My diet became clean, green, and conscious; my intuition became so heightened and at first it freaked me out so much, I thought I could sign up for the next psychic convention as their keynote speaker.

People commented that I looked really, really healthy and glowing, and they couldn't quite put a finger on exactly what it was, but something was different.

Synchronicity was a norm on any given day; there was an effortlessness to my routine that made me feel like I was on an escalator and something else was doing all the work for me. I was moving, but there was no effort involved.

My energy eventually returned, and life as I knew it was never going to be the same again. Crappy situations still happened, and life still went on, but I was becoming more and more resilient to stressful situations. Things didn't stress me out like they did before. I grew stronger and more at peace with the natural unfolding of life.

I was slowing down physically, and as I did that, my intuition ramped up. I was allowing the divine flow of life to move me in the direction I was supposed to go. I have now termed this the Pace of Grace.

The Pace of Grace is about being divinely guided to your true self and able to tune in to a higher vibration. I was being guided the whole way. Intuitively I was awakening to the exact food, supplement, or modality my body needed. As I cleansed toxins and heavy metals out of my system, I also purged years of built-up fears, anxieties, and toxic emotions.

As I did this, I began to realise that I didn't need to struggle in order just to get by. I started to draw back the curtain of lack that had blocked the window of abundance. As old energies were leaving my body, joy had room to enter. Joy began to fill the space where stress had once resided.

A few years ago, if you had told me I would be writing a book on how to slow down in life, I would have laughed my head off. I would have told you that if you want to know how to speed up in life, make things happen quicker, get things done faster, then I'm your girl, but slow down? You've got to be joking.

Life's too short; I'm on a mission, damn it, and time's a-wasting. See, I'm just a girl from the wrong side of the white line who went on a hero's journey very young, slew lots of bad guys, and won the battle.

The white line was the broken line in the middle of a main street that divided our suburbs. On one side was middle-class suburbia; on the other, a housing commission estate nicknamed the ghetto and, you guessed right, I was on the other side.

So I learned to stand up and fight for what I wanted early on. There were no free rides where I came from. If you wanted something, you worked bloody hard or you stole it. Either way, it involved a fierce determination and a certain amount of courage, mixed in with some large balls to get what you wanted.

The fact that I made it out alive, not addicted to drugs or knocked up, was the result of some very well-directed prayers from my grandmother and also a still, small voice that would whisper to me that there is more to life and there is a better way.

The thing is, when you grow up a fighter, life presents you lots of circumstances to fight for. It's like the harder you try, the harder it gets. One step forward and three steps back. That never-give-up attitude is pinned like a medal of honour on your heart.

It's a "screw you" attitude with a little Aussie battler flag flying high on the post. Struggle becomes your middle name, and picking yourself up, dusting yourself off, and getting on with it is just how you roll.

"Suck it up, princess" became my motto, and "Get over it" were the first words I learnt to say.

That is great for those times that call for courage, persistence, and tenacity. When you live like that 24/7, your body has to work twice as hard to maintain the energy. It's like going uphill with the brakes on. You don't get anywhere fast, and then you've worn out the motor before you've made it up the hill.

Eventually, something has to give, and it will, trust me (more on that later). I lived by the notion that if it is to be, it is up to me, and that's a big load to bear. It's a never-ending, constant battle to have to be the only energy that makes life happen for you.

Your environment can harden you and you get tired from trying to prove yourself over and over again.

In my twenties, I created a personal training and therapeutic massage business that became a great lifestyle but never gave me more money than I needed. I was always struggling with money. If I worked three jobs I still wouldn't have any money; it's like the harder I worked the less I had. I might get some spare cash and my car would break down. Something always happened to eat up whatever money I had.

I wouldn't put up my prices because I didn't believe in myself enough to do so. I had a major self-esteem problem. I had a very low sense of self-worth. I was super judgemental and critical of myself.

I was living an unconscious life, I was not nurturing myself, and I didn't love myself. I abused my body with cigarettes, alcohol, sugar, caffeine, and fatty foods. I lost myself in binge drinking.

I was not grateful; I felt as if I lived in lack all the time. I changed who I was to be accepted by others. I didn't even really know who I was. I had childhood hurts and gaping wounds which I ignored, suppressed, and anaesthetised.

I kept my feelings hidden, I was jealous of others, I was envious of the way life just worked for them, and I was scared.

I was not living up to my potential; I dreamed of a life so different than the one I lived.

I was fearless in my work but fearful in the pursuit of my dreams.

I longed for freedom but kept myself caged with the rod of criticism.

I yearned for authenticity and uniqueness but conformed to the masses so as to never experience judgement and humiliation again.

When life is a struggle your body feels struggle. When you're working triple time just to get by your organs work triple time as well.

When you have beliefs that nothing comes easy then nothing comes easy. You deflect effortlessness and ease so it's not even on your radar.

When life threw me curveballs I would analyse it in my head in order to move on; I would put a positive spin on it and tell myself to buckle up and suck it up. My head was very good at moving on; I didn't listen to my body or my feelings because I didn't like the feelings; they made me feel like a victim or a loser.

When you avoid your feelings they get trapped in your body, and cause disease and sickness. They just want to be acknowledged and released. I would wrap them up in my story and keep them suppressed.

What I did have going for me though was a voice that continually whispered that there was a different way and there was more to life. I was tenacious; I had deep-seated longing to be more and I desired more. I had a belief that there was nothing in life I couldn't handle, and I had a curious and open mind. Those traits were my saviour.

My journey with personal growth has been an unfolding: a layer upon layer of gentle yet sometimes obsessive quest for self-discovery. I was born into this world to experience revolutionary transformation. This is not a wimp's journey. I had to become my own hero.

I now call myself a modern day alchemist: I turn the trash of my life into treasure.

The last eight years have taught me a better way to live: more effortless, slower, gentler, nurturing, loving, and kinder. This doesn't mean playing smaller or giving up on my dreams; in fact, my dreams got bigger and I attracted more people into my life.

Adrenal fatigue for me was life's way of saying, okay, it's time to go deeper, and it's time to access a wisdom that cannot be obtained by my previous existence. In the slowing down, I uncovered a pace I never knew existed, a pace talked about in films like *The Secret* and in books like *The Law of Attraction*. To me it was a concept I was yet to grasp, so the Universe showed me how.

There is a StressLess way to live. A way that doesn't prematurely age you, where it unfolds organically and where grace has a chance to shower blessings on you in ways you would have never known before.

The blessings are not necessarily anything new but the miracle is you see them as blessings, not curses. That's where you reduce the stress. It's your perception of what is.

My life changed dramatically during those years; I learned to slow down and simplify. This doesn't mean having less necessarily. What it means is there is a deepening, a shedding, and a letting go, which occurs so that you can align yourself with the flow of life.

The Pace of Grace is in fact the flow of life which unfolds when you are guided by Source; whether it be God, Buddha, the Divine, it doesn't matter what you call it. When we slow down physically, we amp up our intuition, we hear God more clearly. We pay attention; our sixth sense becomes sharper.

It is then you attract what it is you really want. Rather than wanting lots of stuff you get to learn what your soul's desires are. Your world gets bigger and expanded; not in a hurried sense of bedlam and chaos, but a natural organic ease.

I changed my beliefs about certain things. I shed rules that I had adopted years before which were no longer serving me. I was having an internal dialogue with my feelings and they told me secrets that made me hoot, holler, and howl.

I was having a physical shift and a cellular change. I had made friends with stress; my cells were tingling. My nervous system was repairing itself; my adrenal glands were basking in the love.

And the really cool thing, if that wasn't already cool enough, was that my intuition just opened up like a flower in spring. The beautiful still, small whisper was at last being heard again. I was vibrating at a higher frequency so I was attracting circumstances and situations which before were off the radar.

Gradually I was changing my cellular setup which was one of struggle, striving, and lack to one of ease, joy, and abundance. My biology was literally changing as I adopted this new lifestyle.

Marianne Williamson once wrote that our outside world is a reflection of our internal conditioning. What is happening internally is creating the energy that you are.

As I changed physically, mindfully, and spiritually, my outer world shifted in response. In the presence of this peaceful state, I began to get new ideas and new revelations were commonplace.

The verse at the beginning of this chapter says it all:

"There is a way of living in the world that is not here although it seems to be. You do not change your appearance although you smile more frequently, your forehead is serene and your eyes are quiet."
A Course in Miracles

"Your eyes are quiet": that makes me smile. What would your life be like if your eyes were quiet, if you smiled more frequently, and if your forehead was serene?

In this book, I share the practices that I learnt whilst on my sabbatical of wellness. My desire is that you are empowered with choices. I am simply sharing my story and the ways in which I transformed my life. I pray that you become so in tune with your body and with life that you quantum leap right on over to your divine potential. How you do that is up to you; there is no one-size-fits-all here. You can choose to do a couple of my practices or all of them. The more awake you become, the more you will hear what your body is telling you; your soul will whisper where to go and your spirit will keep you safe.

This is a holistic approach to living a StressLess life. My suggestion is to take a lean-into approach: just baby steps. Some of these steps I have been working on for years and years. Yet as we inch our way forward, life sees our progress and rewards us with blessings beyond our wildest imaginings.

If you have fun with these principles they will take you on a dance where unlearning becomes a waltz and remembering a tango.

Be gentle with yourself is wisdom's advice; love yourself through each and every step. Far too often we beat ourselves up with our thoughts. Nothing halts the Pace of Grace more than the energy of self-criticism.

Accept responsibility, surrender into the unknown, let go of control, and let life take you on a journey of discovery more magical than Disneyland, more beautiful than a sunset, and more precious than the rarest diamond.

CHAPTER 2

A Soft Place To Fall

And the winner is ... Enrich Retreat & Spa.

This was one of the best nights of my life. My business, the one I had poured my heart, soul, blood, sweat, and tears into, had just won the award for the best rural day spa in Australasia. After only eight months of operating.

I thought I had succeeded in creating my dream, yet in reality what I had created was a soft place to fall.

Having worked in the corporate world and being co-director with my husband for our training and development company, I knew about stress, and the pressure to perform and conform to company polices.

With the retreat and spa we wanted to create a haven for stressed-out, busy people to retreat, reinvigorate, and nourish themselves. The location was perfect: three acres of sub-tropical rainforest overlooking a beautiful lake; you couldn't ask for much more.

With our lifestyles, we have forgotten what it feels like to be still in our bodies. We think that if we are sitting in front of the TV with our feet up, that is relaxing. Five minutes at the end of the day to have a cuppa and stop moving does not necessarily stimulate the parasympathetic nervous system, which is our rest and relaxation response.

What is happening today is that we are stuck in the fight, flight, or freeze response and our adrenals are continually working overtime, our bodies are producing cortisol, and it is making us sick.

That is what happened to me. For years I got my energy from my adrenals instead of my food. My body was so compromised that my digestive system wasn't able to absorb all the nutrients it needed from the low-quality food I was giving it. My liver was so busy working overtime trying to break down the toxins and poisons in my system that all my energy was just going on that.

I was also in striving mode: there was a pushing energy that I was constantly tapped into. There was no gentle flow down the river; I was paddling upstream with all my effort, making sure that I was achieving my goals, dreaming big, striving for a six-figure business in the first year, winning awards, and being the most attentive wife and friend I could be, amongst other things.

So here I was, creating a beautiful haven for others to relax and un-wind in whilst all the time my body was saying, "It's me you need to be concentrating on."

But that's the thing I totally dig about life: it will give you everything you need to do whatever you are called to do. I said I wanted to help people get back to feeling amazing in their bodies, and so the Universe in all her innate wisdom provided me with exactly what I needed in order to go to a depth that I would never have gone to if it had not been for the adrenal fatigue.

It was one of the greatest teachers I have had, although if you had told me that when I was first diagnosed I would have bitten your head off.

One of the biggest struggles I had to release was the guilt associated with not working all the time. I would be curled up in bed for a nana nap at eleven a.m. because I had absolutely no energy to do anything else, and I would be berating myself and calling myself a lazy so and so. There was no self-love where that was concerned.

I had a work ethic that saw me start work in my uncle's fruit and vegetable shop when I was twelve years old, and since then I have held down usually two jobs at a time. When I went into business for myself and became an entrepreneur, my whole life was my work. I identified with it; it was who I was.

The biggest question I had to ask myself was, "Who am I without my work?" I honestly didn't know the answer.

I see it so much with mothers. Being over-identified with the title of "Mum" and completely losing themselves in the process. We can get so caught up in a label—cancer, diabetes, overweight, depressed—that it takes a leading role in the movie that is our life. You are supposed to be the leading lady or man of your own life, and who you are isn't determined by your circumstances or your diagnosis.

I also prided myself on being independent. I was a self-made girl who was never given a free ride in life and everything I had I got by my own strength. Independence was my freedom. It was my backup plan. I didn't need anyone else in life; I was a survivor.

Now, here I was and I didn't have the energy to cook, clean, or work. I needed my husband and my staff, and I had to admit that and feel okay with it.

I needed to learn that I'm not a failure if I ask for help. People will help; it's in our nature. Yet I felt like I was being a burden, but that gets you nowhere fast.

And the slowing-down thing was so foreign to me. Because I would feel severely overwhelmed, I had to literally just lie down on one of the sun lounges and bask in the sun. It actually sounds really stupid as I write this, but back then that was something I only did on weekends or my days off, never at two p.m. on a Monday.

My mind was thinking I was doing nothing, but what I was actually doing was conscious restoration, and that for me took a lot to get my head around. My body needed to repair itself and the only way to do that was for me to literally stop.

I also couldn't exercise. I am an ex-personal trainer and now my body wasn't physically able to exercise. When you have an injury that literally inhibits your ability to function, you realise how much you take your health for granted. Your body needs all its energy and resources to repair and rejuvenate, so any additional pressure means a longer recuperation time.

Your safe place is where you go to ask the big questions. My whole life was literally being dissected as piece by piece I went deeper into the whole experience. Where did I adopt the belief that I wasn't worthy if I wasn't working? Why is being independent so important to me? Why do I feel like a failure if I'm not sitting at my desk?

These are questions I asked myself every day, and later on I will share with you the formula I used, and how I was able to literally blow any kind of limiting belief out of the water. This process, which was so simple yet profound, eventually enabled me to release the struggle and stress which was keeping me so compromised in every way. As I surrendered into this allowing, my whole body started to relax. The guilt disappeared and I felt myself softening.

I felt like the rigidness that had contained my being for so long was melting into this alchemic liquid that was turning the dross of my life into gold dust.

Eventually I realised I was practising self-love and that was a concept very foreign to me. Yet as I leaned into it and learned to embrace loving myself, I soon realised that there was so much more unfolding than I had thought. I had allowed unapologetic self-love into my life, and this became the mattress for my soft place to fall.

My beautiful retreat was my healing sanctuary as my body and soul renewed itself. While I was healing so too were others who were coming to the retreat. As I took my hands off the wheel, the spa was able to continue to be a place of rest for others—surprise, surprise.

And that is what I learned: when we release the grip on our dream, then the Universe has a chance to do its thing. The grip is our own fears. Control is fear, and once that is surrendered and replaced with faith then we will see divine purpose in play.

Mastin Kipp from *The Daily Love* wrote that grace arrives the moment we decide to let go of what we can't control, focus on what we can control, and let something greater take over.

When our bodies are compromised, dreams and desires take a back seat to just making it through the day. Stress literally imprisons our freedom to dream the big dreams.

I believe in soul dreams, the divine dreams that our soul yearns for. Yet we, as mere mortals, get in our own way and screw up. Take Moses, for instance; they say that for years he walked his people around the mountain because he was too scared to enter into the promised land. A trip that should have taken, say, eleven days took forty years. So we are kind of like Moses in the fact that we let our fears, insecurities, and doubts prevent us from walking into our promised land. Or if we do fight our way through and get to our beautiful promise, then we end up with our legs up the wall in a restorative yoga pose because we don't have the energy now to enjoy it. Bugger!

This is not the end of the road though because grace gets a chance to confetti-bomb us with love.

Life wasn't meant to be this hard. Yes, crappy things happen and we go through unbelievable heartache and grief, but I honestly know in my spirit that we are never given anything we cannot handle. Miracles can appear from absolute devastation when we shift our perception of what is.

I once had a beautiful friend called Nina. We became besties when we were twenty and training to be nurses in country Victoria. Now I'm a country girl, but she was from the sticks. She grew up in a town with a population of no more than one thousand. She was a total good girl with a heart of gold, and her dream was to be a nurse; that was all she ever wanted.

She married her childhood sweetheart when she was only twenty and when we graduated she went to work on the children's ward at St John of God Hospital in Ballarat.

She had her dream man, her dream job, and a smile you couldn't wipe from her face. Then one night she didn't show up for her shift at work. After a couple of hours the staff called her parents. Her father and younger brother thought it was really strange so they drove the five minutes it took to get to her house. It was there they found her body, unrecognisable. She had been bashed and left to die on the front veranda of her home. They have never found her killer.

The whole town showed up for her funeral; they had to have speakers scattered around the gardens so the people who couldn't fit in the church could hear her service.

I don't know why that happened. If I ask why, all it does is take me down a path of despair and heartache. I choose to shift my perception and focus on how she lived her life. How she had the courage to live her dreams. We don't know how long we are called to live this life; I figure if I'm going to live it fully then I want to do it with energy to spare at the end of the day, with an extra shot of mojo to keep me going. I'm going to plan to go the distance but know that any day could be my last. So with that in mind I am going to live like every day is special, treat my body with such respect so that it can go the distance with as much vibrancy, spark, and juice as I can muster.

That is my dream for you. I want to see your dreams actualised, see you reach your divine potential and living your inspired purpose. Where circumstances and situations don't knock you out of the game. Where health issues do not limit and contain your greatness.

That is the reason for this book, the reason why I took the time to write it. This is my love letter to you. This is my divine purpose, to help you reach your highest potential. This is the reason the Universe gifted me my soft place to fall. So I could slow down long enough, so I could hear the still, small voice, raise my intuition, and together we could create change in the world in our lifetime. However long we are here on this beautiful planet we call home.

Hopefully you read this book before you are so stressed out that burnout is your body's only option. In saying that, if you know that you are heading down the path of stress, struggle, and fatigue, and that life is giving you warning signals, then you're going to need a soft place to fall. A place where you can go slower than you've ever gone, in order to go deeper than you've ever been. But you don't need to go out and start a spa and retreat in order to find that place.

All you need is the permission to give yourself unapologetic self-love and a space in your heart for it to take up residence.

Unapologetic means not feeling guilty when you take time out for yourself. It means not apologising for putting yourself first on occasion. It also means having the courage to make the changes you need to in order to live a StressLess life.

If this concept makes you clench your butt cheeks at the thought, then it is exactly what you need. You can't give to those you love when your tank is empty. You have to give from your overflow, meaning you do the things that fill you up first, and then what you give to others contains far more joy and love than it would had you given from a place of exhaustion and overwhelm.

Living a StressLess life is a gift you give to yourself; it transpires over time. Each time you work on yourself you unwrap a layer of the gift wrapping. Every time you enter your soft place you get to realise just how amazing this gift is.

I am not saying that it's all champagne and roses; it's a lot of effort at times. At times you will want to tell life to take this gift and shove it where the sun don't shine. But if you're reading this book, I'll bet that the magnetic pull of the promise of a life full of ease, joy, and abundance will prevent you from doing that.

I'll bet you have that still, small voice inside you whispering that there is a better way, an easier way. That voice won't go away, no matter how much you push it down with alcohol, drugs, sugar, or work. Life wants to show you what grace feels like. It wants to unveil all of its wisdom and beauty to you. There is abundance available to all who seek it. There really is a joy, which is palpable. And the way to get them is effortless once you enter your soft place; rest on your mattress of unapologetic self-love and tap into the Pace of Grace.

CHAPTER 3

Stress: Your Biggest Block To Intuition, Abundant Health and Desires.

As a traveller on this planet, living in the fast-food, fast-paced, ASAP rat race we all call life, I've come to realise just how much our supercharged lifestyle affects us.

We've gone for bigger, better, faster, louder, taller, and stronger, but all we have achieved is we've gotten busier, sicker, and fatter and we end up burnt out, stressed out, maxed out, and then we check out.

Life becomes dull; we lose the colour, the sparkle, the essence, and joy goes out the window. We walk around living unconscious lives, lost in a world of disbelief and fear.

Fear, anxiety, stress, and tension constrict us; we literally vibrate at a denser energy, which blankets our intuition. It deflects wisdom, creativity, and the body's ability to heal.

How do we navigate this thing called life in such a way as to reduce the effect that stress has on our lives? How do we live our full potential, achieve our greatest dreams and desires, and rock our worlds, all without getting sick and deflecting the wonderful law of attraction?

How do we tap into the heartbeat of life, and travel along with ease and grace as our travelling companions?

This book includes ancient wisdom, philosophies, principles, and strategies, which will help you to live a StressLess life in this wild, crazy world in which we inhabit. They will help you to view stress differently, teach you how to go at the Pace of Grace, and how to connect to your inner guidance system. We become so tuned into our bodies that we know the second we go off course, and we can track back to where we are meant to be.

This book is about a holistic approach to reducing stress, struggle, and fatigue and the move in to ease, joy, and abundance. By addressing spirituality, our mindset, energy, and the physical aspect of stress, we can start to radically transform our lives. Miracles happen, grace unfolds all around us, the clouds part, rainbows appear, and life as we know it is radically changed forever.

If we were to look at what stress does to us, it is not only one of the biggest contributors to disease, illness, premature ageing, and death, it is also one of the biggest sabotages of our success.

It literally blocks the flow of our energy, our passion, and our creative genius, and smothers the life force within us. Not to mention making us feel like crap. Yet the choices we make every day continue to contribute to this because we either don't know about it, don't know what to do about it, or don't give a rat's ass about it.

Stress is your response to circumstances. Everyone is different. How you respond is different. What is the same is, if we view stress as bad and ignore it or push it under the table, she will eventually scream, shout, kick, and punch until you sit down and share your lunch with her and find out what she really wants you to know.

What we ingest in our mouths, on our bodies, via our thoughts, in our homes, our environment: it all builds up over time, and one day you wake up and you feel stuck, you feel unwell, you're not happy, life is hard.

I have firsthand experience with this crappy feeling on many levels, and one particular story comes to mind.

Paris, nineteenth of November 2005. I'm standing in a bathroom, too small to swing a cat in, although why anyone would want to swing a cat is beyond me, but now you at least get the picture.

I stare at my reflection in the mirror and take a deep breath. "This is it," I say to myself. I look at the wedding dress hanging on the back of the door. It's an off-white, satin and beaded dress, plain and under-stated, with none of the frills and spills that sometimes accompany the dream dress of a girl's BIG day.

But nonetheless this is my chosen dress for my BIG day, and it had to travel halfway around the world in a suitcase and not get creased, so my choices were somewhat limited.

I slip it over my head, adjust my bits and pieces, and give myself a wink and a smile. I'm about to elope in the most romantic city in the world.

I walk out into our rabbit warren of a motel room, all angles and small corners, and see my future husband sitting on the bed in his freshly ironed white shirt and black pants. He looks beautiful and my heart starts to beat really, really fast all of a sudden. I can see by the sweat on his brow that his heart has been beating that way for some time and I ask him if he has taken his blood pressure medication.

He appears more nervous than I and I figure it would be just my luck that I have to rush him off to the hospital before I get a chance to call myself a married woman and check out of club "singledom". I'm thirty-seven years old, for goodness sake; if it doesn't happen now I'm really going to give up.

But no, he assures me that he is fine and asks me if I'm ready to do this. Am I ready? Yes, yes, I finally am.

I share this with you because my life was about to be completely turned upside down and boy, was I in for one hell of a ride.

Ian and I had been doing the long-distance thing for nine months before we eloped: he in Sydney and me in country Victoria. It made sense for me to relocate to Sydney as Ian's two children lived there, so

I gave up my business, said good-bye to my friends and family, and took my little dog off to the big smoke.

Now here I am, a country girl living in the city with a brand-new husband who I had been dating for only nine months. All of a sudden I am a stepmother to an eight- and eleven-year-old. I have left my business behind, and Ian and I intend on joining forces. I will be partnering him in his training and development company. In what capacity, I have no idea yet; all I know is that his ex-wife is his personal assistant—interesting, yes?

On top of all this, I have no friends, I get lost every time I go out in the car, I hate busy roads, and his parents are coming to meet me for the first time.

I was experiencing so many emotions every day: excitement at being married to the man I love, sadness at leaving my friends and family, loneliness and isolation, fear when driving on the Sydney roads, doubt as to where I fit into his kids' life, and, if I was honest, jealousy because his ex talked to him more times in a day than I did. I could switch back and forth between these and numerous other emotions in a nanosecond.

To say I was stressed was an understatement. My health was starting to decline. My energy, which was once unstoppable, felt like molasses in my body. My allergies were on the attack and my weight was on the rise. I was making really unenlightened choices, to say the least. By this time in my life I had been a student of personal growth for over ten years, but you wouldn't have known it judging by the emotions I was experiencing and my response to them. I had completely shut down my intuition so I was being ruled by ego and fear.

In addition to this, I started to feel like a tile on the wall. Before, I had always been fuelled by my desires and they burned with a combination of tenacity, hope, and ass-kicking mojo. Now, the stress of my life had distinguished my fuel and the only thing happening to my middle aged ass was that it was dropping fast.

See, that's the thing with life: there are always going to be situations and circumstances that are out of our control and we need to get through them the healthiest way possible. In today's fast-paced, busy lifestyle we can be so focused on just making it through the day that we feel we don't have time to slow down and deal with what is actually causing the stress. The longer we ignore it, though, the worse it gets.

When we get like this our bodies internally respond to the outside external forces. Hormones become unbalanced, toxins are released, muscles contract, organs constrict, systems shut down, cells atrophy, the ageing process is sped up, our bodies become fatter, our arteries become restricted, cells mutate, and we call it getting older.

We ignore the signs and symptoms; we go to the doctor who pre-scribes drugs to make us feel better. We get diagnoses like cancer, heart disease, diabetes, or however it happens to manifest for you.

And it doesn't just affect us physically: emotionally we suffer; we lose the spark, the fire. Our passion goes out the window. We do what we do to get by and that's all the energy we have to give. There is sad-ness, an undercurrent of heaviness. Life is singing the blues and we can't seem to change the station. We may end up getting diagnosed as depressed and are advised to take antidepressants.

Our intuition goes out the window; we no longer feel or trust our sixth sense. It's like a cloud has descended upon us and our navigation system is shot. We seem to be flying blind. We deflect the law of at-traction so it is not even on the radar.

The longer we ignore the silent urgings the more intense these symp-toms get. It's time to stop ignoring what is stressing you: slow down physically so that you can slow down internally, hear the still, small voice, ramp up your intuition, and get on with what your soul has called you to do.

The longer we let stress, struggle, and fatigue lead our lives, the longer we delay our desires.

So, back to my story: my life had changed so much that I needed to take a pause, and reassess where I was and where I was going. Firstly, I needed to learn what being a wife meant, as this was all new to me. I was still figuring out his bathroom noises.

I then had to figure out where I fitted into an already-prepared family. I knew the kids didn't need another mother, but what did they need from me and what did I need?

Then there was the issue with my business. Starting a business with a partner is one thing, but coming into an already existing setup and saying, "What can I add to this partnership?" when I had existing issues around self-worth and needing to feel equal just adds an extra dynamic into the scheme of things.

It was like my past collided with my present and all of my fears and sabotaging beliefs came flooding out. I was forced to deal with parts of my childhood that I had kept locked up.

There was a part of me that felt like an outsider my whole life, and then I ended up in a family where once again I felt like an outsider. Like, come on, Karina, let's deal with this once and for all.

They say that relationships will reflect our crap right back at us, and I had four beautiful souls (including the ex) reflecting my crap back at me and it was not pretty.

No matter where you are at in life, no matter what your stress may be, if you just allow yourself to go slower than you've ever gone, in order to go deeper than you've ever been, you will experience the magic that is the Pace of Grace.

So I slowed down enough to let my body breathe. I allowed my internal system to realign itself again in order to find that beautiful, natural balance and alignment.

Then I went deep enough to heal and to forgive. I travelled back into the deepest depths of my being, and through the tears and the pain came the transformation and the breakthrough.

It is with delight that as I write this, Ian and I are coming up to our fifteen-year anniversary. Our businesses continue to change and grow, and I wouldn't want any other business partner, even if Richard Branson were to personally come and invite me to go into business with him. (Well, maybe if it was Richard Branson.)

I'm not saying it was easy, but I am assuring you it was worth it. That is what life is about; it wants us to succeed and be the greatest version of ourselves possible. And that is why I chose to write this book and share the steps to achieving a StressLess life. So that we can all travel through life with ease and joy in our hearts. So we can get through the tough times with greater resilience and strength. And in the unburdening of ourselves, we become liberated, healed and whole.

CHAPTER 4

Make Stress Your New BFF!

It's a controversial title, I know, but stick with me and hear me out for a sec.

We all know what stress is and how it affects us. There is the good stress that prepares us to go into battle, and then there is the bad stress. In this book when I refer to stress I am referring to the chronic kind. It is the ongoing fight or flight response that leaves us stressed out, burnt out, maxed out, and eventually checked out.

The view of most people is that stress is a bad thing. But what if we took a different view? What if we said that stress could be a positive thing when we change our view on it?

In a TED talk by Kelly McGonigal, titled "How to make stress your friend", (https://www.youtube.com/watch?v=RcGyVTAoXEU) she stated a study by Keller, Litzelman, Wisk et al. 2012, University of Wisconsin, School of Medicare and Public Health tracked thirty thousand adults in the US for eight years. They asked people how much stress they had experienced in the last year. They also asked, "Do you believe that stress is harmful for your health?"

Then they used public death records to find out who died. People who experienced a lot of stress in the previous year had a 42 percent increase risk of dying ONLY if they had the belief that stress is harmful to your health.

People who experienced a lot of stress but didn't see it as harmful were no more likely to die. In fact they had the lowest risk of dying than anyone in the study including people who had relatively little stress.

Over the eight years, one hundred and eighty-two thousand Americans died prematurely not from stress but from the belief that stress was bad for you: that's twenty thousand people a year.

Can changing how you think about stress make you healthier? The science says yes. When you change your mind about stress you can change your body's response to stress.

Let's look at chronic stress as anything that puts a strain on our life. Strain that leads to pressure, inflammation, disease, and illness, both physically and emotionally.

What we ingest in our mouths, on our bodies, in our homes, our environment, all builds up over time. One day you wake up and you feel stuck, you feel unwell, you're not happy, and life is hard.

Stress also results from a negative thought. When we think the same thought over and over again it becomes a belief. Change your thoughts and you can literally eliminate the stress associated with that thought.

Early on in my childhood I had a number of experiences where I came to the belief that life was not safe. Over time, additional experiences where trust was broken by someone in authority to me cemented that belief into my cellular structure. When we operate from this dynamic we are essentially living with an open trust wound.

Physical wounds that don't heal can eventually lead to loss of limbs or loss of life. Metaphorically speaking, anybody walking around with a gaping, unhealed trust wound will never be able to fully experience their divine potential because they have become cut off from receiving the full power of Source.

Constant thoughts about not feeling safe caused me to try and control everything. This need to try and control the outcome of certain events and situations led to pressure and strain on my internal system.

When we can't trust that life has our back and that everything is working out to our highest and greatest good, we manipulate life, essentially pinching ourselves off from our life force.

I felt I needed to make things happen myself because I didn't believe that life loved me. When I couldn't force the outcome to my liking, the more I resisted and persisted. This way of living kept me stuck in my sympathetic nervous system. My adrenals were overworked and cortisol was coursing through my body.

The thing is, I wasn't even aware of this; I was so disconnected from myself that it felt like it was my normal state of being. I missed the signs that were always there, warning me that things were not balanced.

Signs which included suppressing emotional moments of deep sadness and hurt after I had failed to achieve a goal I was working so hard for. Bathing in regret for not listening to my intuition and following up on that lead that could have been highly beneficial for me. Getting stuck being overwhelmed at the thought of having to do everything myself, yet never asking for help. Blaming myself for failed toxic relationships.

Our soul cries out in order to be heard over the constant jackhammer-like torture we put it through every day. For me this looked like the constant criticism which I directed at myself for not being good enough. The abuse I heaped on my body by not nourishing it with wholesome food, and by ingesting poisonous toxic chemicals every day, like alcohol and cigarettes. The act of judging everything I did and never feeling like I was worthy of praise. The blame, shame, and guilt I wore like a yoke around my neck because I thought that was what I deserved.

The emotions and feelings are always there; we just need to get good at hearing them. Then we need to know what to do when they do show up and how to release them in a healthy way.

Let's take the example of a tsunami. A tsunami is not a good thing, yet we can now predict when one is coming. There are signs, and these signs are a good thing. People can prepare and do everything in their power to stay safe.

The same thing applies for stress. Stress is a series of signs in our body that tell us we think something is not right. Usually we think it's not right because it doesn't feel good. We focus on the feeling or emotion, naming it stress and labelling it as bad.

Instead of looking at this as a negative we can change our thinking. We can view it as a friend that has something important to tell us.

We can become still for a moment, and become aware of our thoughts and the sensations in our body. Are these thoughts serving our higher selves or are they hoodwinking us? Are these sensations pleasant or do they feel like pressure?

Then we can go deeper and look at what our body is trying to tell us. This is the ultimate in mind-body connection. The tightness in our chest, the muscle pain, the headaches, the fatigue and exhaustion: they are all there to lead us to our highest version of ourselves.

Stress, acting as our dear friend, only has our best interest at heart. She is there to warn us that maybe we shouldn't be eating all those donuts because we're putting too much stress on our arteries and heart with all that chemical-laden fat being pumped around our body.

She is there to warn you that those fears you have of not being enough, of not feeling worthy, are actually producing acid in your body which is affecting your internal organs and speeding up the ageing process.

She is there to warn you that all those hours you're putting in at work, trying to have a bigger house, a nicer car, the latest iPhone, is causing you dis-ease because what your soul really wants is to take that art course and spend more time with your family.

When you are not in alignment with the Pace of Grace, your fears and insecurities hurt, they cause pain. When you are in alignment, they have no trigger; you can observe them without emotion.

Stress is a cover or a label for the feelings underneath that you don't want to acknowledge. Allow yourself to feel the feeling without the story behind it and you will ease the stress. Then you become empowered and can do something about it.

Stress can become your greatest ally if you use it to navigate forward. When you understand it, it will tell you what to do when pain, disease, fear, or discomfort is on the playing field.

Stress is simply your response to circumstances based on your thoughts and beliefs. Everyone is different. How you respond is different to someone else. What is the same is that if we view stress as bad and ignore it, or push it under the table, she will become the stalker from hell and turn into your own worst enemy.

It is the story you associate with that causes the emotion. We often get lost in the story of a painful situation only to heighten the feelings. These feelings intensify, and the stress in our body causes the blood to run to our arms and legs, leaving our head. So with little blood flow to our brains we go into stupid mode. Reasoning leaves us behind. Creativity has left the building.

The possibility of making mature, rational decisions goes out the window. This is when we drunk dial or post messages on Facebook we just know we're going to regret later.

A good friend wouldn't let you do that. A good friend would intervene somehow. And that is what stress is being. She is being a good friend. She is the racing heart whilst you're speed dialling. The nausea before you hit post. The thing is, we are not listening; we are too caught up in the story to hear her.

I made friends with my stress a long time ago. I even have a name for her; she is my StressLess Sage. She saved my life countless times. Let me share her story.

If you said that I was ambitious, driven, and an overachiever, then you would be correct. I believed that if you worked hard you could achieve anything. Life never came easy for me, even as a kid. Everything was a struggle, but that made me even more determined to push against the odds. I was a fighter, and I guess that work ethic made me appreciate everything I had achieved so much more.

My family lived in a housing commission area and we were known as the westies. People would lock their doors and roll up their windows if they ever had to drive through. Most of my friends were on drugs or pregnant by the time they were sixteen. What stopped me going down that path was a small voice inside me that kept whispering, "There's more to life" and "There is a better way". The voice, which I now call my StressLess Sage, saved my life and she still does today.

I've been involved in health and wellness throughout my whole career. After training as a nurse and working in the public health system for a few years, I kind of figured that all I was doing was treating the symptoms and not the cause of the issue. I realised I was focused on the disease, not the wellbeing of a person. I felt conflicted, and would lie awake at night and wonder if this really was what I was meant to be doing, and I would feel the passion for something I worked so hard for slowly leave my body. Sage kept speaking to me: "There's more to life, there's another way", so I listened and was guided down a different path.

I then decided that I would try and keep people healthy, so I became a personal trainer and holistic massage therapist. I loved this work because I saw some real results and breakthroughs.

I was a tough-love kind of trainer; you know the type: no pain, no gain, suck it up princess, and if you vomit that's great. No excuse was good enough for not completing your program. The nutrition program I was taught to provide was loads of animal protein, salads, vegetables, and dairy. Frozen meals were fine, I said, and go for the low-fat, diet-food variety. That's pretty healthy, most people would think. We were certainly trained to believe that the food pyramid was the Holy Grail.

The problem was I was drawn to natural alternative therapies, and the more I learnt about this new world, the more I realised a lot of what I was taught just wasn't true. I was feeling like there was an integrity gap in my life, and this is a quick way to cause stress in your body.

Then Sage spoke her magic words again: "There's another way, and there's a better way", so I went down another path. I opened a day spa and retreat called enRich Retreat & Spa and we focused on deep rest and restoration. I knew that so many people were not putting themselves first and with our stressful lives to-day, disease and ill health is a major issue.

We focused on an organic vegetarian diet: lots of raw, delicious foods and green juices. We eliminated toxins and chemicals from our cleaning products, and also the products we used on ourselves. We grew some of our food and looked after ourselves with natural alternatives, instead of prescribed medications.

Sage was leading me down the path of a StressLess life and the more I followed this path, the richer my life became. I started to see how stress affects every part of our lives. My eyes were opened to what stress is and how I dealt with it.

Given my very ambitious nature I made it my goal to have an award-winning spa, and within eight months of opening that dream came true and enRich Retreat & Spa won best rural day spa in Australasia. The thing was, I was so focused on the high of achieving the goals, I wasn't paying attention to the everyday miracles that were occurring in my life. Just how far I had come from the young girl who thought she was "less than" because she lived on the other side of the broken white line. The teenager who rebelled against authority because people in authority had hurt her more than words could say. The young woman who struggled in business every day because she knew no other way.

I had alchemised my life to the point where it was no longer recognisable, yet I wasn't seeing that. I was blinded to that miracle. All I saw was the miracle of winning an award and gaining my self-worth through what I did, not who I was. "There's more to life, there's another way": Sage was back.

After that, my body said enough and I was diagnosed with stage-two adrenal fatigue. I then had to stop for a while. If you're not listening to your inner sage, life will gift you with something where you will be forced to stop.

The big thing for me was the guilt I felt because I couldn't work. Sage told me that stress comes in many forms, and our negative thoughts and feelings are one of the biggest toxic contributors to the body. Stress literally dims your lights, boxes you in, and contains your greatness.

Over the next twenty-four months, Sage introduced me to many principles, tools, and philosophies on how to live a Stress-Less life. I had no choice but to listen, and through this process I healed myself and the StressLess Revolution was born.

There is another path that you could follow where you practise personal mastery, where you could become the healthiest, most energetic, vibrant, and effervescent version of yourself imaginable.

There is a StressLess path where you can have all of your dreams and desires with more depth and meaningfulness imaginable.

So next time you are feeling overwhelmed or stress of any kind, take a moment and check in with yourself. Ask yourself what thoughts you are thinking. What sensations are you feeling? Listen to Sage's sweet voice and be guided to a higher awareness.

Get out your journal and start to write down everything you are feeling. Breathe into the awareness and know that you are safe. Sage is there to protect you. There is something you must pay attention to in order to live a StressLess life. Hold space for insight and healing to occur for it is in the healing that the revealing of your Soul's Highest Expression (SHE) will transpire. SHE will lead you on a journey filled with more passion, more love, and more beauty than you can ever imagine. It will feel like the sun, moon, and stars come out to shine just for you.

Life has your back, I know that now. I can trust that no matter what occurs in life there is nothing that I cannot handle. I can gaze into a sunset and be healed from wounds that I once thought were so deep and incurable, now seen as a gift in the form of a divine teacher.

The more you listen to the StressLess Sage and pay attention, the easier it will be to access the Pace of Grace. The more times you enter a safe place with Sage by your side, the less stress you will have in your life. Watch out, one day you will open your beautiful eyes and see that you are now living a StressLess life.

CHAPTER 5

Slow Is The New ASAP

When you get off the rat race and onto the path less travelled, life becomes a whole lot deeper and more meaningful. Circumstances and coincidences happen more frequently. Chance meetings with the person that can open the right doors aren't so "chance" anymore.

The slow-down-to-speed-up philosophy is not about doing less or taking a longer time to do things. It's like when you get on the travelator at the airport. You stop walking and let it do the work for you. It becomes effortless. There is less struggle and resistance.

It's like finding life's pulse and getting in the perfect groove. In order to find this, you first have to slow down and listen for the beat. In our fast-paced lifestyles we can't hear what life is telling us. What our bodies are trying to let us know. We ignore the signals and before we know it, we've got cancer or heart disease or diabetes.

The forty-fourth verse of the Tao Te Ching by Lao-tzu says, "Know when to stop, if the chase is wearing out your health, stop. If the chase is wreaking havoc on your relationship, stop. Exhausting you, stop. When you know when to cease and desist you are protected from all the perils and you will enjoy a long and contented existence."

The chase is the constant wanting and striving for more. The not knowing when to stop is the cancer that is killing us.

All it takes is a few minutes a day to breathe and hear the whisper. "Don't feed me milk anymore, it makes me sick inside" sounds like cramping and bloating. "I'm scared of failing" sounds like tightness in the chest. However your body talks to you, it is trying to have a conversation with you all the time, but you won't hear it if you're not taking the time to be still and listen.

The more we pay attention to life, the louder the heartbeat and the closer to the groove we get. We attract our desires quicker because we are not in the way. We are going with life's flow and not against it. The more we allow life to unfold organically, the more blessings we receive. The more we slow down and listen, the more grace has a chance to unfold in our lives.

Slowing down means adopting a simpler life, but not in the terms of playing smaller, necessarily. As a matter of fact, the simpler the lifestyle I adopted, the more profound my life became.

There is a depth that you can attain when life becomes simple; there is a connection to all living things that becomes so strong it's almost palpable. Peace and joy become the norm.

Simple embodies a softness which the Tao Te Ching says overrides the hardest of all things.

I believe "simple" can be found in many variations and forms. As I continue my energy-clearing work and release past hurts and fears, my cellular structure restores itself. There is a simplicity found in the awesomeness of one's natural state. The removal of blockages allows for the chi or energy to flow freely through and around our bodies. The more blockages we have the more complex and complicated our lives become.

Another form of "simple" is found in the food we eat. The closer to its natural source, the higher the life force. The more processed it is, the more complex the ingredient list is on the back of the packaging.

Complex food leads to dis-ease in our bodies. Dis-ease in our bodies leads to complications in our health.

The accumulation of "stuff"—the need to fill our lives up with "more", the unwillingness to let go of things—leads us away from simplicity street and stuck in complicated court.

Simple goes hand in hand with ease. It allows room for a breath. It creates a cavity for grace to play in. In this space we let go of the "push, push" energy and take hold of a "divine pull" that lifts us up and carries us along.

This "divine pull" is like a magnetic force shield, a cosmic dance that takes place once we slow down long enough to feel the rhythm.

It's like the cosmos is offering you a free ride; you just need to sit back and trust it. The only effort you need to exert is the effort required for you to slow down. The rest is effortless.

The result is you become more productive; you think clearer. You are far more creative; you attract all that you need into your life. You lose the perception of chronological time and shift to eternal time. This time frame knows not of minutes or hours, it only knows of simple vibration. It is not about reaching your goals this year or in three to five years' time. It can happen in an instant the moment we let go of the struggle, stress, and fatigue, and tap into the Pace of Grace.

My husband loves acronyms so together we came up with one for this chapter. F.A.S.T.E.R. It's a guide on how to get to where we need to be faster by actually slowing down.

The "F" stands for Flow not Force

My husband, Ian, was trying to lock down a meeting with a person who he thought would be instrumental in getting one of our company initiatives off the ground. Try as he may, this person was being elusive. No matter what he did he continued to get the brush-off. After a while Ian became frustrated that it was taking so long and he was starting to get disheartened that it may never happen.

One day, on a walk with our dogs, I explained that I felt there was this forced contraction in his energy, a tightness around his body when he talked about this person. When we hold onto something so tight we don't allow any room for God to do His thing; it's like we squeeze the life right out of it.

We did a process called tapping or Emotional Freedom Technique: EFT. I use this process all the time for clearing blocked energy from the past and de-stressing. I talk about it at length in chapter 15.

At the start of the tapping his anxiety around this situation was a 7.8 out of 10. As we tapped he started to relax to where he felt no anxiety whatsoever. Exactly two and a half hours later, the secretary of the woman whom Ian had tried for months to get a meeting with emailed and asked if he was available for a meeting that Wednesday at one p.m.

All we did was take all of the forceful energy away from the situation, which allowed a flow effect to come in and take over.

There is a difference between doing all that you can to make something happen and forcing it to happen. It comes down to the emotion and energy behind the action. Force has an emotion of fear around it; flow has an energy of trust and surrender.

Fear constricts and vibrates at a lower frequency than trust or surrender. Law of attraction operates to the frequency you are vibrating at. When we choose our desires and attach fear what we get is a lot of complicated setback. If we attach faith that says "this or something better" and surrender from the outcome, we can come into alignment with the "divine pull", which in turn leads us to the best possible results.

The "A" stands for Attract don't Advertise

Anyone in business knows that advertising can cost an arm and a leg. In the beginning of starting up the day spa, I spent thousands on advertising in papers and magazines. I remember we ran an advertisement in the local paper and cancelled our lunch date with friends because we had to sit by the phone to answer all of the calls that would come in. We didn't receive one call.

Now, advertising can work for some businesses and there are many places to advertise but what we eventually found out was attraction is a whole lot cheaper and easier.

That's why it's called the law of attraction, not the law of advertising. It's free. There is no need to make something look better than it is. There is no call for discounts or bright shiny lights.

Attraction works by being completely and utterly authentic. Simplicity is its calling card, effortlessness its landing page.

The "S" stands for Slow not Stressed

When we are stressed our bodies go on heightened alert. Our hearts race, our pulses quicken, blood pressure rises, adrenals go on full alert, and cortisol is released throughout the body. All the body's defence systems are preparing to go into fight, flight, or freeze. There is major activity going on and this is happening continually throughout the day.

Chronic stress is when our bodies are in an allostatic overload and cannot achieve homeostasis. We cannot attain to a natural state of well-being.

When we slow down long enough to allow awareness to dwell within the tissues and cells of our bodies, we become in tune with this imbalance. We sense that hormonally and chemically we are out of alignment, and we are intuitively led down the path to our healing.

Our bodies tell us what we need; they talk to us all the time. If we can just listen with the ears of unapologetic love for ourselves we would choose differently. Stress would give way to wisdom, which would carry us forward into a new era of nurturing and self-care.

The "T" is for Tapped In not Tuned Out

Abraham Hicks talks about this all the time: being tuned in to our bodies. This is what slowing down is all about. It allows us to sense exactly what it is we need to do to get to where we need to be faster.

When our bodies are compromised by too many toxins and chemicals, our organs need to focus all their energy on trying to repair and restore. There is no room left for thriving. Dreams take a back seat to just making it through the day. We literally cannot find the station we need to tune in to because there is too much white noise and static in the way.

When our minds are so scattered, focused on the past or the future and not grounded in the here and now, trying to tap into our guidance system is a total failure. It is like trying to find a program on channel ten when the television is tuned into channel seven. It just ain't gonna happen.

By taking the time to restore the body, focusing on the thoughts we are thinking and accessing a higher power, we can tap into the Pace of

Grace. Our intuition becomes amplified, our life force magnified, and divine potential actualised.

The "E" is for Ease not Effort

There is a difference between ease and easy. We all experience times when something is easy. No effort required and no resistance experienced. When someone is travelling at the Pace of Grace, life is not always easy but there is an ease associated with it.

Does this mean that there won't be hard times, loss, sorrow, or pain? No. Does it mean that you won't have to work in order to achieve your desires? No. Does it mean that you will get everything you want? No.

By now you're probably asking, well, just what does it mean, Karina?

It means finding the graceful way through. It means your effort is spent on achieving effortlessness. We must all go through hardship at some point in order to grow. We must all experience loss because that is what it means to be human. We cannot get everything we want, but I promise you will get everything you need.

The secret is to find the ease through the dis-ease, the comfort through the discomfort, and the heart in the heartache. It's there if you look; ease will reveal itself with the unfolding of a miracle. The unravelling of a silver lining, and the revealing of a lesson learnt. Ease will soothe the brokenness of a heart by the practice of gratitude. It will look like compassion and feel like forgiveness.

Ease will sometimes seem like the hardest thing to find, yet if you so desire, it will find you. Ease won't always be easy, it may not necessarily be effortless. But it is always there, waiting for you to choose it.

The "R" is for Restore not Resign

Resigning isn't the same as surrendering. Resigning feels like you've lost, like you are a victim. It's a defeatist attitude. Surrendering means releasing the attachment to an outcome with a knowing that what will be is for the highest good. It's not a no, it's a not now. It's a comma not a full stop. It's this or something better.

When we resign ourselves to something it usually means we have given up and accepted what is. I see a lot of people who have resigned themselves to their particular illness or circumstance in life.

When I was diagnosed with adrenal fatigue and heavy metal toxicity, I could have resigned myself to the fact that I am always going to be tired and feel like I've been run over by a truck.

Instead, I resolved to restore my body to its natural state, to do everything in my power to get well. Restoration is bringing something back to life, resigning is like a death. When we restore we infuse vitality, we embed charisma and soul. In order to speed up your desires, you need to restore your life with these characteristics.

This ASAP model of life that we have chosen to make our mantra doesn't seem to be working for us. The way I see it, it has cheated us out of experiencing absolute wellness, the frustrating delectableness of delayed gratification, and the joy of knowing divine potential.

I think it's time we realised slow is the new ASAP and adopted the F.A.S.T.E.R. approach to slowing down, in order to speed up.

CHAPTER 6

Benefit From The Selah Effect!

Selah means to pause; it's often used in the old biblical hymns at the end of a verse or before an amen. It's what we do in the "pause" of our lives that determines the greatness of our success.

If we never used commas in our sentences we would be left with a string of words all running together and not really making sense. Selah is the comma in our lives; it's a chance to breathe. It's in this pause that we get to do the things that make our hearts sing and our souls dance with joy. It's also in this pause where we get to dissolve a lifetime of hurts and fears in order to release our greatest potential.

I call it conscious downtime. It's planned, it's thoughtful and, if need be, scheduled. It's a soulful blend of inner dialogue, reflection, dreaming, and activities which nourish the spirit.

When our souls are fed then creativity can flourish, ideas come effortlessly, and energy flows freely. Problems are solved without stress, the law of attraction works in abundance, and you get to shine your brightest light to the world.

Selah is a chance to love yourself by being kind and respectful to yourself. It's a chance to get to know the real you, how your body talks to you, what thoughts go through your head.

What it is not is five minutes with your feet up at the end of the day, coffee in one hand and trashy magazine in the other. This is called checking out, my friend, not tuning in.

Selah is also the conversation you have with your inner child, the one you put off having because it could be painful. There could be tears and discomfort. As a matter of fact, there most likely will be sometimes, but there will also be so much joy and peace mixed in that it makes it worth it.

You go slower than you've ever gone to go deeper than you've ever been and that eventually leads to a depth of peace, which sadly not many people experience unless they have the courage to go there.

Three years after opening the day spa I realised that my soul was longing to journey down another path. This book you are reading was longing to be birthed and I was being carried along by the "divine pull" to go deeper than I've ever gone.

My energies were being torn in too many directions and I was becoming overwhelmed again. I kept being drawn back to a conversation I had with my astrologist, Lisa Zimmerman. She told me that my career would not come from my work but from my transformation.

At the time, whilst I had renewed my adrenals, I found out that I had seven times the amount of aluminium and arsenic in my system, as well as a couple of other heavy metals thrown in for good measure. I was determined to detox my system as I knew that aluminium overload was a precursor to diseases such as Parkinson's, Alzheimer's and dementia.

Lisa's words just kept coming back into my spirit and I remember vividly her saying to me, "You created an award-winning business, can you create an award-winning you?"

I looked around my beautiful retreat and in my spirit I knew it was time to move on. It was time to concentrate full-time on being the best version of myself possible. So with much gratitude and love in my heart, I packed up my award-winning business and started to devote all my time into loving myself unconditionally.

I was going to take an extended "selah", for however long it took. A pause in my career in order to gift myself something I had never been able to give: pure, unapologetic love and respect.

All my life I believed my self-worth came from what I did; if I wasn't succeeding in my work then I was a failure. When we believe our value comes from things outside of ourselves, or letters after our name or even being a parent, we greatly diminish the magnitude of this gift called life.

Material things will come and go; you will find no lasting joy in spending your years attaining a bigger house or the latest car. There will always be something more to have.

What we do is a significant part of our life but it doesn't define who we are unless we let it. A cleaner in a school has as much value as the prime minister. I have seen people retire one day only to have a stroke on the golf course the next because their whole identity is wrapped up in their work, and without that they don't know who they are.

Children are a gift given to us so we can raise them into hopefully becoming functional, contributing adults. Yet so many women lose themselves in motherhood, only to wake up twenty years later as an empty nester with no idea of who they are.

I had to find my value from "who" I was and "who" I was being, and when I did that years of pain and heartache slipped away. The moment I released the shame over not reaching all my business goals or making my yearly forecasted revenue, my soul did a happy dance. Handing the keys over to the spa meant freedom.

It was only in the selah moments that I could hear the still, small whisper. It was only when I slowed down that the divine pull could latch on. In the pause of our life soul expressions have time to marinate. Life takes on a softness and a new depth of flavour that wasn't previously tasted.

Major life decisions are debated and deliberated on with the help of some universal wisdom and divine insight. Creativity is allowed to run free producing brand-new ideas that are exactly what you needed. Clarity and certainty are invited onto the playing field.

In the forty-third verse of the Tao Te Ching by Lao-tzu it says, "The softest of all things override the hardest of all things." It encourages us to become like water: soft with the ability to enter everywhere.

Selah is about becoming soft. Releasing the rigidness and hard lines from your life and surrendering into the smoothness that is the Stress-Less life. It's a chance to breathe out all of the forcing energy.

You can't hold water by grabbing it; instead, you have to relax and open your hand. And so it is with life: the more you relax and let life work for you the simpler life will become. Tasks will become easier; relationships with others will be peaceful. Hard-and-fast rules melt into 'soft and slow', making way for miracles to unfold.

The moment you relax and stop pushing, you can become like water and find yourself in spaces where normally you couldn't get to. Dreams and desires you have held in your hand for so long are now lapping at your feet like the waves of the ocean. You've softened enough to allow them into your life.

The more often you practise selah moments the softer life gets. Now I find ways to make everything a selah moment.

If I am writing I have incense and candles and meditate before I start. When I am cooking I have music on in the background to relax me. If I am cleaning, my energy is towards loving on my home, not focused on it being a chore. The exercise I do now is focused on slowing down my system; long walks in nature and yoga provide the replenishment my body needs.

If I need to read something or do research, I do it in one of my al-chemic baths. It is here I get the insights and intuition that lead me to my biggest ideas.

There are many ways we can do the mundane and boring things in life without getting stressed or thinking negative thoughts whilst we do them.

Just as there are ways to go through the layers of your life without it causing heartache and more pain.

After selling the spa and moving house I felt really disconnected from Source. I decided to take a soulcation, which is basically selah on a holiday, a soulcation is a vacation for the soul; clever, hey?

We sat down together, my soul and I, and I asked her what she wanted to do, and she proceeded to give me her rules:

1. Any activity we do has to be soul enriching
2. No gossip mags, TV or mind-numbing movies
3. Food has to be clean, green and conscious, and raw chocolate was very much allowed
4. Rest when needed; loads of sleep is a priority
5. Alchemy baths are a necessity
6. Loads of personal space and alone time is a non-negotiable
7. We must connect with nature every day
8. This time is all about unapologetic self-love

Okay, awesome, this sounds like fun, I told her.

Well, anyway, here is a brief rundown on how my week panned out:

Monday:
Slept in, yummy. Meditated, prayed, soaked in the tub with my Doterra oils. Walked the dogs. Made my green smoothies, loads of yummy salads, and raw chocolate treats. Watched a course on opening up the higher chakras with Carol Tuttle, totally loved this content. Listened to some recordings from the Food Revolution Summit with John and Ocean Robbins.

Tuesday:
Woke up early and watched the sun come up over the valley. Meditated, prayed, did some yoga on Gaiam TV, ate yummy green food. Burnt lots of incense. Did an hour of Feldenkrais, stretching; my back loved it. Watched some videos from the Hay House World Summit. Did some more on my higher chakra course. Took a nap after lunch. Lit the fire at night and sat with my dogs cuddled up, feeling the love.

Wednesday:
More of the same except this time I did my Soulprint healing work which is an online course through Mindvalley with Carol Tuttle. It is all about healing your soul through energy work. I highly recommend it if you are into that sort of thing or at least open-minded. I am experiencing huge breakthroughs.

Thursday:
Bought an energy medicine kit by Donna Eden. If you haven't heard of Donna she is an awesome energy healer, and has a lot of really practical energy techniques to open your chakras and clear subtle energy blocks. Also listened to a recording with Anthony Williams from the Hay House World Summit who said that being present in the moment at sunset helps to clear trust wounds so I have made watching the sun go down part of my daily activity. Listened to Doreen Virtue's meditation for affluence and wealth in my alchemy bath.

Friday:
Informed my husband that I was rewriting our soul contract for marriage. He thought I had been smoking something. But our souls have contracts and we can rewrite them at any time if we want to. Our last nine years has included a lot of struggle and lack so we decided to go into our tenth year with the energy of ease, joy and affluence. Look out world, here we come.

Saturday:
Market day today: lots of fresh, organic, soul-enriching food. Home to cook up a heap of veggie delights for the week. Cleaned up our wellness area of our new home which includes a meditation room, gym, infrared sauna, and hydrotherapy spa. Tried some funky Ganesh dancing on Gaiam TV; definitely got my groove on then.

Sunday:
Cleaned the house whilst listening to Sade, saged the house as
well. Relaxed in the sauna and spa. Listened to some more recordings, watched some more Hay House movies, had a nap, and
did some meditation under the stars.

Well, that was pretty much my week. My benefits included
(but were not limited to):
- Overall feeling of joy and peace
- Much more balanced and centred, inspired insights and
  clarity for my work
- More connected with God
- Shed one kilogram – wasn't trying to but it just re-
  leased from my body
- So much more relaxed
- My body felt soft and I had lost that contraction be-
  tween my shoulder blades
- I felt excited to be getting back to work

After that week, I went to work on this book you're reading with so
much more ease, insight, and inspiration than if I had have just pushed
straight on after moving house. You may think that you don't have the
time to take a soulcation or even meditate for fifteen minutes a day, but
Gay Hendricks in his book *The Big Leap* talks about Einstein time. How
time is not outside of ourselves, it is actually within us.

We make as much time as we need and if you can get your head
around that concept, then it makes sense that by slowing down in order
to come back to our natural state of being, we are not a victim of time
but rather the creator of time.

What we achieve when we are in alignment is far more powerful and
divinely guided than when our bodies are stressed out.

In yoga there is a posture called Savasana or the corpse pose. It allows the body time to process information it has received. Selah is like
the Savasana in your life. It is the essential ingredient needed when living a StressLess life.

I encourage you to make "selah" a regular part of your life, to schedule it in the diary if you have to. It is only when you do this that you can begin to know what the Pace of Grace feels like. It is only when you go deep that life begins to take on a depth and breadth you never knew existed. When you have the courage to step up and be a spirit warrior, let your fears, your pain body, and your shadow self step into the light, you illuminate the darkness. You transcend the ordinary struggle, stress, and strain of life and revolutionary transformation can occur.

CHAPTER 7

Amplifying Your Intuition With The StressLess Cleanse

I totally believe there is no one-size-fits-all: no one diet works for everyone; no one exercise program is suited to all bodies; no one form of StressLess living is the right fit for every person. That is why my goal is to help you release the blocks from your intuition so that you can know what is right for your body.

Stress blocks us from hearing the guidance our bodies and senses are sending to us. We either don't hear it, ignore it, misunderstand it, or refuse to listen to it. But in order to live a StressLess life and tune into the Pace of Grace we have to pay attention to the signposts along the way, and those signposts are our intuition pointing us in the right direction.

When we are living life in the rat race, so consumed with going along at the pace we push ourselves at, we miss the pace that life wants us to live. If we actually slowed down long enough we would see that this pace is slower and quieter. The white noise is removed and what is left is a peaceful melody.

All of a sudden we know intuitively what move we need to make next, who to contact, what to say no to, and what to say yes to. Whereas before there may have been confusion attached to this inner guidance, now it is clear and bright. The fog has lifted; no longer are we letting negative emotions, fearful thoughts, toxicity, inflammation, or fatigue cloud our intuitive power.

No longer do we suppress the quiet whispers with sugar, push down the inner nudges with an endless to-do list, or camouflage the truth with phantom stress.

The more blocks we remove caused by stress, the more we move into our natural state of being. Each time we lean a little more into the StressLess lifestyle, we lessen the grip of struggle, stress, and strain. Every time we travel at the Pace of Grace our vibration rises. When this happens we access more of our intuition. We tap into a higher consciousness and it is from this place where a new depth of living arises.

I love eating the food I eat but I know not everyone is going to adopt this lifestyle. I do, however, think it is essential that in order for you to clear away the blocks to intuition, you need to cleanse regularly. If you have been eating a high-processed, meat-heavy diet, your system has probably been under some stress for quite some time in order to digest and eliminate the toxins, chemicals, and preservatives found in a lot of food lately.

It needs a rest, my dear; it needs a reprieve from the onslaught and time to cleanse itself, and start to realign back to its natural state. From here our organs have a chance to repair themselves; our systems have the opportunity to function at optimal performance again.

Cleansing is not dieting; I don't believe in diets. I think by eating a wholefoods, organic, plant-based diet we can achieve all the nutrients the body needs in order to maintain homeostasis. By cleansing we are eliminating certain foods which inflame the body and cause it to work overtime. We also eliminate environmental toxicity. This allows the cells to become healthy again so that they can actually absorb the nutrients we are ingesting.

When I started to change my diet and drink my smoothies and add all the goodness back in, my body was so compromised that it couldn't actually take in all the nutrients I was supplying it. I needed to regenerate in order to rejuvenate.

I tried a number of different cleanses, detoxes, and fasts, and what I found was the more processed my diet was to begin with, the harder it was to complete the cleanse. The detoxification process was a lot more intense because there were so many toxins being released. After about day three, I started to feel so much better: I wasn't hungry, I had more energy, and my mind was clearer. This is where intuition starts to heighten.

The cleaner my diet was on a regular daily basis, the longer and deeper I could go into a cleanse. So I am suggesting two choices. Choice A is a seven-day juice and smoothie fast where all you consume are green juices, teas, smoothies, and water. You may choose this option if you don't have the time to commit to a full month of cleansing or if you think that it would be too much of a stretch for you to start with.

Choice B is a twenty-eight-day vegan and raw food cleanse. On this cleanse I found that I didn't go hungry and there were not a lot of side effects due to the detoxification. By the end of this month I felt the healthiest I had felt in years.

Now I make cleansing a regular part of my yearly program and aim to do at least three to four fasts or cleanses a year. If I try and coincide them with the start of the seasons it makes it easier.

Choice A: Seven-day fast

This cleanse is best done by having green juices for the first half of the day, and green smoothies in the afternoon and evening. The juices are easier on your digestive system which aids in digestion, and the smoothies contain the fibre and are more filling sustaining you through the later part of the day when we usually eat more. Include water with lemon and also water with green powder such as spirulina. This helps with the detox symptoms, which may include headaches, muscle aches, diarrhoea, or nausea. Herbal teas are also allowed but make sure they are decaffeinated.

You can have as many juices as you like throughout the day but make sure you stick with green fruit and vegetables, such as celery, cucumber, kale, chard, spinach, green apples, and limes.

I loved the movie *Fat, Sick, and Nearly Dead* with Joe Cross. Joe was overweight and sick. He decided to do a juice fast for sixty days across America. He now has a mini-empire online. You can watch the movie free at http://www.rebootwithjoe.com/watch-fat-sick-and-nearly-dead/ if you want added inspiration and motivation.

Also Kris Carr from www.kriscarr.com is a great resource for juices and smoothies.

Choice B: Twenty-eight-day cleanse

To make it simple, you start off with one week of going vegan, eliminating all meat, dairy, and animal products from your diet. The coffee and alcohol needs to be put on hold for the complete cleanse as well; sorry, guys, but I promise your body will love you for it, and it's not a not ever, just a not now. The next week is all raw foods—nothing cooked above forty degrees Celsius. Week three is a green juice and smoothie week, but if you can't go a whole week on liquid only, go as long as you can and then switch back to raw foods, or do a combination. The last week is back to vegan.

In her book, *Soak your Nuts – Cleansing with Karyn*, 2011 Book Publishing Company, Karyn Calabrese provides a detailed twenty-eight-day cleanse which she calls nature's healing system. I highly recommend this book as I have found it is a gentle approach to restoring our bodies back to their natural state. A word of advice, though; if you are not in the US, you may find it difficult to get a lot of her supplements she recommends, but you can find alternatives in your health food store which have the same effect.

I found the main thing is to be organised and plan ahead. I have my four weeks of meals all planned out. Then I do a shop and stock the pantry. There are so many awesome vegan and raw food websites around now so I just get online and look for recipes that are easy to make and that I know my husband will enjoy too.

After the first cleanse the others are easy because you have all the recipes and shopping lists you need. If you tried a recipe you didn't like then just replace it with something else. I find it is all about trial and error. There are also some great recipes for cleansing on my website at www.karinastephens.com so make sure you check them out as well.

Body presence

In addition to cleansing your body an important tool I use for amplifying my intuition is body presence. Tuning into how our bodies are feeling a few times every day will enliven us to greater presence and insight.

Sit quietly and allow a few deep breaths. Bring your focus inwards and start to scan your body, starting with your toes and moving all the way up to the top of the head. Notice for any tightness, constriction, or any other sensations. Do not make any judgements; just notice it and move on.

Once we are present and have connected to our bodies internally we move our attention to our power centre, which is located about three inches below the navel and in the middle of our bodies.

In a body of work called *The Art of Feminine Presence* by Rachael Jayne Groover, she calls this space for women the womb space. This is the area in which the womb takes residence, or would take residence if you have had it removed. For men, it's a dude space.

With your eyes closed, bring your awareness to this space in your body; imagine your pelvis area and contained in this area is a bowl taking up all the space. In the bowl is a beautiful light globe, illuminating and warm. This is your home space, your power centre, and when you are connected here you are home, as Rachael Jayne would say.

Once you have connected to your power centre, bring your attention up to your heart. Breathe into your heart and imagine it breathing back; feel warmth surrounding this area, and feel the connection between your heart and your power centre.

Now imagine a golden rod running through the top of your head, right through the middle of your body, connecting all of the chakras. This rod comes from heaven and into the earth, grounding you. This is your vertical energetic core. You want to energetically lean back into this space. It is not at the front of your body; it is back into the middle, and by leaning back and feeling the rod aligning all the way through the middle of your vertical core you can really get the sense that when you lean back you are right on it.

This is where you are most present; you are strong and grounded, connected to the infinite power of the divine and grounded strong into mother earth. This is your place of authenticity and power. This is where you can access your intuition from a place of knowing and certainty.

The more you practise being in your vertical energetic core and operating from this place, the stronger your intuition will be.

Intuitive chakra

The intuitive chakra is known as the sixth chakra and is positioned in the middle of the forehead, so it is called the third eye. Its colour is indigo and it represents intuition and psychic talents, self-reflection, visualisation, discernment, and trust of your own intuition.

Fully opening up this chakra will enable you to really switch on your intuition. Below is an intuitive chakra opening meditation; you can access the recording at www.karinastephens.com/pog-gifts

Intuitive chakra opening meditation

Close your eyes and imagine yourself standing in a beautiful light, being bathed in the warmth and feeling safe and secure.

Imagine a shaft of light coming down from heaven entering into the top of your head and activating your crown chakra. Notice your crown chakra opening up like a beautiful purple lotus, allowing the shaft of light to enter down into the middle of your forehead.

Now see this light filling up the front and back of your head, and opening up your third eye. See your eye literally open its eyelid and a beautiful indigo colour appear.

Take a deep breath and see that your eye is facing inwards; this is your inner vision or insight. Now see a beam of light coming out of your third eye and projecting outwards, lighting your path with inner knowing.

Say out loud, "It is safe to trust my intuition. It is safe to receive guidance and I trust that what I see and feel is the truth."

Now, allow a deep breath and come back to where you are sitting; slowly open your eyes and know that you can do this meditation whenever you want to.

So these are a couple of ways in which I amplify my intuition and really live life at the Pace of Grace. I am not second-guessing myself; I don't regret decisions I have made. There is a peace which comes from operating life living in the know. Being able to trust yourself and being comfortable with that is a great way to live the StressLess life.

CHAPTER 8

The StressLess Kitchen

Part One: Superfoods

Welcome to the StressLess kitchen. This kitchen is unlike most kitchens you come across. This is where magic happens, where "trying" to be healthy is an oxymoron because there is no trying here, there just is.

This is where we shed rules, restrictions, and constrictions and begin an adventure where curiosity is our magic carpet. There are no latest-fad diets, no one telling you to eat at certain times whilst standing on your head facing north. This time it's all about you and your biology; you are the creator of what you eat in the StressLess kitchen.

You were born hardwired to know exactly what is needed for your own body and soul to thrive. It is in each of our DNA, a blueprint of success, and all we have to do is recognise what it feels like to remember what our body needs, and all this takes place in the StressLess kitchen.

What has happened is that our bodies have been so compromised with synthetic foods, chemicals, toxins, preservatives, additives, and a host of other unnatural substances that we have created a thick fog of forgetfulness, blanketing our cells. In order for us to remember how to eat for longevity, we need to remove the fog.

The plan for most people is to add more years to their life, right? We want to live as long as we can, and we are actually succeeding in this. The issue is we are not living longer but we are dying longer. The quality of our existence is being compromised by disease and illness, which society calls a natural ageing process. Well, I say boohoo to that; there is enough scientific evidence today that will back up the belief that if we drastically reduce or illuminate certain additives to our diet we can avoid falling victim to these hideous illnesses.

I want to add more years to my life, but I want to add more life to those years, and that is the key ingredient in the StressLess kitchen. How do we firstly restore our bodies back to their natural state, detoxifying from a synthetic food system, and then not only rebuild but transform our entire body into a living, breathing expression of divine perfection at any age?

Well, that is what this chapter is all about, so if you're interested, stick around.

Firstly, we are going to take all the stress out. It is no use having a StressLess kitchen if all you are is stressed because you can't have your coffee in the morning, or your beer at night. All I am suggesting is that you add certain superfoods and superherbs into your diet. Then look for a natural source for your other foods, meaning choose a food that is not processed to the hilt and has so many numbers in the ingredients that it resembles a math test.

There is so much hype out there about avoiding certain foods, such as those containing gluten, and if you have conditions such as coeliac disease or gluten intolerance then by all means stick to what your medical advisors are teaching you, but what I want to point out is that food is not the enemy. Wheat is not the enemy here. It is what we do with the wheat: how we break it down, process all the goodness out of it, add in toxic preservatives that is the real issue. Choosing bread, which is a wholefood organic source of real food, is what I am suggesting. Buying wholegrain pasta instead of white processed pasta, choosing a natural sweetener instead of processed white sugar.

We want to choose the foods which have come from the earth and have had the least amount of altering. It is when we alter them so far from their natural state that they begin to cause the biggest amount of stress on our bodies. This is why we are getting the allergies, the ailments and the diseases—not from the food source but from the altering.

So that is all I am asking you to change: choose a food which is closest to its natural state, not a toxic mimic, and then add superfoods and superior herbs to your diet. Easy, hey?

What happens when you do this is that your biology will lead you to your medicine. You've heard the saying: "Let thy food be thy medicine and thy medicine be thy food"? Well, essentially what the StressLess kitchen is doing is enabling your original medicine to be brought forward and presented to the world. This is unique to you and that is why there is not one diet for everyone. Your body is so beautifully handcrafted: every cell, every mitochondria, every atom is perfectly one of a kind. You intuitively know what you need to eat in order to thrive, and it is in the remembering of this that the alchemy happens. The relationship and communication which develops not only between you and your body but your body's organs and systems is truly enchanting. You begin to understand the language your body speaks to you in. Your internal organs start to communicate with each other again, responding to their needs and co-operating together instead of competing.

Eventually your biology will be in charge of what you eat based on your hardwiring and your soul's higher purpose. That's right, I said your soul's higher purpose. The saying "You are what you eat" has been around forever because it is a universal law. When your body is provided with nutrients, which assist it to thrive, your energy vibrates at a higher frequency. When this happens the light in you grows. The light is your soul—your spirit, if you prefer.

My friend Mason Taylor from Superfeast explains it so wonderfully. He uses the analogy of a candle. Your body is the wax; it needs to be strong and grounded and supported in order for the candle to function and fulfil its purpose. The wick is your Qi, or your energy. This relates to the energy in your body, how much vitality and life force you have.

The flame is your Shen, or your spirit: the brighter the flame, the higher your connection is to the divine.

The StressLess kitchen works with these three entities. We build up your body, helping it to become strong. We add in superfoods to the diet, allowing it to restore itself to its natural state again. We work on your Jing energy, which is your primordial life force energy. By consuming Jing herbs, tonics, and elixirs we create a seed bank or a reserve of energy to keep you functioning at your optimal performance. Then we look at superior herbs, which relate directly to your Qi, the energy you use to get by on a daily basis. You want this energy to be high so that you have a spring in your step, bounce in your body, and pep in your stride no matter what your age. Now we focus on the Shen superior herbs; we look at how we can make your light shine brightest, bringing forth your potential and unlocking desires and dreams, which are your birthright.

The StressLess kitchen is in two parts: the first part provides an overview of what superfoods are and how to incorporate them into your diet. The second looks at superior herbs and building up your life force. Before we go further into this chapter I want to address the issue of stress on our animals and livestock as it is an important part of creating a StressLess planet.

If we think about it, a lot of us are eating the diet our parents fed us when we were young. I, like most Australians, was raised on a diet of meat and three veg, those vegetables being potatoes, peas, and the occasional side of lettuce.

Every weekend we would sit down to a treat meal of fish and chips from the corner shop. Soft drink and cordial were staples and Mum's lolly jar was forever being filled up.

I had so much sugar in my diet I ended up with thirteen amalgam fillings in my teeth which I have since had removed.

In my twenties my diet became mostly reliant on fast food and Kraft mac 'n' cheese. I dabbled with being a vegetarian but all I did was give up meat and consume more bread and pasta. Not good if you want healthy, glowing skin.

In my thirties I started to become more conscious of nutrition, the result of completing my personal training certification. We were taught the basic food pyramid and preached protein, protein, protein. As I became busier I stocked the freezer with Lean Cuisine meals and ate from the microwave.

I never thought about the animals I ate, I never read the back of the box, and I never considered how my diet was related to my consciousness.

Basically my food choices were chosen based on my upbringing, what my parents ate. It's funny how I rebelled against everything else but what I put in my stomach.

Eating animals is not something I consciously chose to do, it was inherited, and for the majority of people it is the unquestionable norm. Below is an excerpt from an article on the www.animalsaustralia.org.au website. With their permission I have included information about the state of the food industry in Australia, and how we can begin to make personal choices and empower our lives.

"Industrialised animal abuse hidden away in factory farms and slaughterhouses has become the **single greatest cause of animal cruelty** today. Yet no one asked our permission. We weren't even told there was a choice to be made".

Every day, more people start to question this situation. And the great news is: it's never too late to make a difference. You're about to discover how to take back your power, and make truly informed choices that are in line with your own values.

The humble act of grocery shopping is our most powerful opportunity to vote against animal cruelty. Every time you shop, there are important decisions to make:

Factory farms still exist because unwitting shoppers purchase their products. If you disagree with confining intelligent pigs in crates so small they can't turn around; or performing surgical procedures on animals without pain relief, then the choice is simple: **join the growing number of Australians who** refuse to buy factory farmed products.

Find the meat-free section of the supermarket and try out some exciting new foods! Opting for cruelty free alternatives is the single best way to ensure that farm animals — who have been *excluded* from critical animal cruelty laws in Australia — are protected from abuse.

Think twice about eggs. Most egg-laying hens are forced to spend their short lives crammed inside battery cages where they can't even stretch their wings. **Avoiding cage eggs is crucial**, but laying hens in *all* production systems are killed when their egg production wanes — years before their natural life expectancy. And only female chicks can produce eggs, so millions of unwanted male chicks are gassed or ground up alive each year. This is why many animal lovers are choosing to go egg free.

Consider your milk. For lots of people, it comes as a surprise to realise that cows don't automatically produce milk. Like all mammals, cows only lactate after giving birth. Dairy cows are impregnated each year, and their newborn calves are taken so milk can be harvested for human consumption. Around 700,000 unwanted Australian dairy calves are slaughtered each year at only a few days old as 'waste products' of the dairy industry. So it's not surprising that soymilks, oat milks, rice milks and other delicious dairy alternatives are rapidly gaining popularity among caring consumers."

Initially I became a vegetarian for health reasons; the cleaner my body became, the more my consciousness expanded. As this process was taking place my heart just opened up and became so sensitive to the cruelty of our animals. Personally, I had to step up and be a voice for the voiceless.

If I was going to practise living a StressLess life then that needed to include the animals and the planet at large. I couldn't contain it to just me. My vision became larger and in my dreams I saw a nation of mindful people awakening to what was really going on, and making a stand against big business and governments who continue to practise cruelty to animals, genetically modify, and add hidden toxins in our food.

Vani Hari is the food babe: in her book, *The Food Babe Way: Break Free from Hidden Toxins in your Food and Lose Weight,* she states that we have been duped. "Every bite of food that passes through our lips and every glass of water we drink are potential sources of toxic chemicals, including pesticide residue, preservatives, artificial flavours and colourings, addicting sugars and fats, genetically modified organisms, and more. These toxins can travel to and settle into all the organs of your body, particularly the liver, kidneys, gastrointestinal tract and lungs – and do great damage."

Her website www.foodbabe.com is an amazing wealth of knowledge and she is a powerhouse when it comes to getting big business to buck up and remove dangerous toxins from their food, or at least put it on their labels.

Vani also states that scientists are now realising that chemical-laden food is a major reason why obesity, heart disease, chronic fatigue syndrome, infertility, dementia, mental illness, and more are all on the rise.

Is there any wonder our internal bodies are so stressed out? How can we align ourselves with our natural state when everything we put into our mouths is unnatural?

So even if you are not prepared to become a vegie head or give up your Macca's then please look out for sources of meats which are organic, or at least the non-hormone, grass-fed variety. Choose organic and cage-free, eggs, try meat-free Mondays; there are so many organisations participating in this program now. Reduce the amount of takeaway you are eating or look for a healthier alternative, like sumo salads or some of the healthier options off the Subway menu. Start reading the backs of labels and opt for a less-processed version.

Now for some fun: I am going to show you how to add superfoods to your diet. Even if all you change is this then you are going to be miles ahead in becoming a healthier, StressLess version of yourself.

David Wolfe is an expert when it comes to superfoods and in his book, *Superfoods: The Food and Medicine of the Future,* he lists his top ten foods which he believes are the most potent, super-concentrated, and nutrient-rich foods on the planet. This book is like the superfood bible and I recommend you grab a copy for your StressLess kitchen. I completed David's online raw nutrition certification and his knowledge in this area is phenomenal.

In this chapter I am going to give you an overview of seven of these foods and show you how you can add them into your daily diet, improving your health beyond your wildest dreams.

Goji berries

The goji berry has a combination of therapeutic actions on the body, otherwise known as an adaptogen. Adaptogens strengthen and invigorate the system, helping people to deal with stress more easily by supporting the adrenal glands.

In Chinese medicine the goji berry is known to harmonise and increase the Jing energy of the adrenals and kidneys, which is crucial for anyone suffering from fatigue or burnout.

They increase the immune function, increase alkalinity, provide liver protection, and deliver anti-ageing compounds, not to mention an assortment of additional superhero qualities.

Goji berries are perhaps the world's greatest longevity food as they have been known to increase the amount of Human Growth Hormone (HGH), which puts this little berry at the top of my list.

How to add them to your diet

Consuming a handful of dried goji berries each day adds about fifteen to forty-five grams to your daily intake. Just chew them; they taste amazing.

You can also make tea, soup or wine with them.

Add them to a trail mix.

Blend them up finely and add them in your raw desserts.

Blend them in smoothies, juices and elixirs.

They make great jams.

They can be soaked and rehydrated with the water being used as beverage or a base for soup stock.

Cacao

Oh, glorious, wonderful chocolate: let me count the ways. The raw cacao bean is one of nature's most fantastic superfoods. It is the best natural food source for many nutrients including antioxidants, magnesium, iron, chromium, manganese, zinc, vitamin C, and omega-6 fatty acids.

Now, note to all chocoholics out there: this does not include our regular supermarket varieties. You want to look for raw organic cacao products including beans with the skin, without the skin, cacao nibs, powder butter, and paste.

How to add them to your diet

Add them into your favourite beverage including coconut water, teas, smoothies, and nut milks.

Sprinkle nibs on your favourite desserts instead of chocolate chips.

Eat them raw as a snack food in a trail mix.

Include powder in any of your desserts.

Maca

They say maca is an acquired taste; I absolutely love it, I could just smell it all day. It is a member of the cruciferous family of plants, which includes cabbage, cauliflower, broccoli, and kale. Maca is a powerful strength and stamina enhancer; like the goji berry it is an adaptogen. It is also a wonderful libido-enhancing superfood.

Maca has been known to improve conditions such as:

Anaemia

Chronic fatigue

Depression

Stress tension

Menopausal symptoms.

It contains five times more protein and four times more fibre than our humble potato.

How to add it to your diet

Maca is generally purchased as a dried raw, organic root powder. Add it to smoothies, teas, nut milks, salad dressings, or any beverage you can think of.

Spirulina

Spirulina is known as the protein queen and belongs to a class of single-celled, blue-green spiral algae. The green colour is derived from chlorophyll and the blue colour is from the pigment phycocyanin.

Spirulina is an algae superfood that consists of 65-71 percent protein which is the highest concentration of protein found in any food. It is classed as a complete protein source and is an abundant natural source of chlorophyll, salts, phytonutrients, and enzymes.

When looking to buy spirulina choose certified organic and make sure it has a "fresh" smell. Avoid the brands that use tableting agents, which help to keep it from crumbling. It should naturally cling to itself.

How to add it to your diet

It can be added to juices, smoothies, water, salad dressings, desserts, dips, and even sprinkled on salads.

Aloe vera

The gel of the aloe vera contains vitamins A, C, and E as well as the minerals calcium, sulphur, zinc, magnesium, chromium, and selenium. It is also chock-full of antioxidants, fibre, enzymes, and polysaccharides.

It has a lubricating effect on the joints, brain, nervous system, and the skin. It is awesome for weight loss and fitness and keeping you flexible and limber throughout your life.

When purchasing, look for the organic variety. Select fresh leaves in preference to bottled aloe vera. Select leaves that are thick with gel and free from white speckles.

How to add it to your diet

The gel is best when filleted, and separated from the leaf with your knife. Once you have removed the gel you can add it to smoothies, elixirs, salads, or salsas. Any food you can think of, really.

You can also use the gel as a moisturising lotion, suntan lotion, or salve for minor burns.

I use it as a face mask although some varieties do have a slight smell which you need to adjust to when keeping it on your face for twenty minutes.

Hempseed

The hempseed is a complete protein source. The oil has the highest percentage of essential fatty acids of nearly any seed on earth.

Hemp body care and clothing is a huge industry now, including hemp paper, rope, plastics, and building materials.

In terms of average nutrient content, shelled hempseed is 35 percent protein, 47 percent fat, and 12 percent carbohydrate.

It contains all the essential amino acids and essential fatty acids necessary to maintain human life. It is far more readily absorbed than animal protein because it blends easily with water, beverages, and smoothies without heat.

How to add it to your diet

There are so many hemp products on the market today such as butter, ice cream, salad dressings, breads, beer, and protein bars. You can eat them alone or sprinkled on salads, or even make your own hemp milk.

Coconuts

Did you know that young coconut water is nearly identical to human blood plasma, making it a universal donor? Apparently during the Pacific battles in World War II, both sides siphoned directly from the coconut to give emergency plasma transfusions to wounded soldiers.

Coconuts are healthiest in their youth when the meat is soft. They consist of 90-plus percent of raw saturated fat. Unlike long-chain saturated animal fats, the saturated fat in coconut oil is in the form of medium-chain fatty acids (MCFA), which support the immune system, the thyroid gland, the nervous system, and the skin. They increase metabolism, which aids in weight loss and supports cardiovascular health.

How to add it to your diet

Coconut flesh can be added to water and blended making coconut milk.

It can be dried or dehydrated with herbs and spices and prepared like beef jerky. Blend it in desserts and ice creams. The cream can be consumed straight up or added to beverages. Add it to curries and other dishes.

Use it to cook with; it is the most stable of all oils when cooked at high temperatures.

So there you have it: seven amazing superfoods which you can add to your diet right now in order to increase your life force, decrease the stress on your systems, and start to feel amazing energy straight away. Your body needs you to look after it; why would you not give yourself amazing living foods so that you can be the best version of yourself ever?

Don't forget to head on over to www.karinastephens.com and check out some of the great recipes and resources available for living a StressLess diet.

CHAPTER 9

The StressLess Kitchen

Part Two: Magnifying your life-force with superior herbs

Remember our candle example in the previous chapter in relation to the wax being our Jing energy: the wick is likened to the Qi energy and the light from the flame is our Shen or spirit? It was actually Daoist master Sung Jin Park who termed them the three treasures.

In an article from http://www.chinese.cn, August 24, 2009, titled "The theory of Jing, Qi and Shen", it states the following:

"Jing has been called the 'superior ultimate' treasure, even though in a healthy, glowing body, the quantity is small. Jing existed before the body existed, and this Jing enters the body tissues and becomes the root of our body. When we keep Jing within our body, our body can be vigorous. If a person cares for the cavity of Jing, and does not hurt it recklessly, it is very easy to enjoy a life of great longevity. Without Jing energy, we cannot live.

Qi is the invisible life force, which enables the body to think and perform voluntary movement. The power of Qi can be seen in the power that enables a person to move and live. It can be seen in the movement of energy in the cosmos and in all other movements and changes. Coming from heaven into the body through the nose (yang gate) and mouth (yin gate), it circulates through the twelve meridians to nourish and preserve the inner organs.

Shen energy is similar to the English meaning of the words 'mind' and 'spirit'. It is developed by the combination of Jing and Qi energy. When these two treasures are in balance, the mind is strong, the spirit is great, the emotions are under control and the body is strong and healthy. But it is very difficult to expect a sound mind to be cultivated without sound Jing and Qi. An old proverb says that 'a sound mind lives in a sound body'. When cultivated, Shen will bring peace of mind.

When we develop Jing, we get a large amount of Qi automatically. When we have a large amount of Qi, we will also have strong Shen, and we will become bright and glowing as a holy man."

Following on from part one of the StressLess kitchen, we now delve into superior herbs. Shennong, the legendary ruler of China who is credited with developing the Chinese herbal system thousands of years ago, described the tonic herbs like this: "The herbs of the Superior Class are the rulers. They control the maintenance of life and correspond to Heaven."

The tonic herbs have unique qualities that make them different from all other herbs. The single most important quality is that they contain an abundance of one or more of the three treasures, *Jing*, *qi* and/or *Shen*. That is why Shennong says that they "supplement the energies and nutrients circulating in the body and prolong the years of life without ageing."

Firstly, I want to explain to you what it feels like to be depleted of the three treasures. At the very peak of my adrenal fatigue, I remember one morning in particular: I had gone to bed at eight p.m. the night before, exhausted. When my alarm went off at seven a.m., I literally groaned out loud. My eyes were as heavy as lead and I could barely manage to open them and turn off the alarm. My head felt so heavy against the pillow that I couldn't even lift it. My body was more than fatigued; I was literally enervated beyond words.

As I looked out my bedroom window I saw the sun beaming down on the lake; I saw the birds in the trees and the bamboo tree gently swaying in the breeze. It was an amazing day and yet as I lay there thinking of all the things I had to get done that day, I just broke into tears, I was so overwhelmed. There was no strength in me to even move past the thoughts; there was no solidity in my being to even begin to talk myself through this. Lying there on that particular morning, I was at the furtherest point from the highest expression of myself. I had depleted my three treasures to the point where there was just but a trickle of compromised life-force left. There was no Qi energy available to get me through the basic daily tasks. I had no passion, no will, no desire to dream any dreams. I had no light; my Shen had dried up.

After I had detoxed my body, I began to incorporate a lot of the three treasure foods into my diet. I needed to build up my life force, and I have to say that it was the superfoods and superior herbs that have brought me back to an even greater level of health than I had previously. Below is an overview of the herbs that I have added into my diet. Mainly I add them to a herbal tonic made with tea; I also use them in soups and desserts. As you lean into the world of tonic herbs you will find a brand-new level of ultimate wellness opening up to you. I encourage you to explore this new world with curiosity and see it as an adventure. Just as with superfoods, superior herbs are the secret for having a StressLess kitchen and living a StressLess life.

It is vitally important that you purchase only the best quality herbs, which from my research you can safely purchase from the following websites.

www.superfeast.com.au if you live in Australia is a wonderful site for purchasing the best brands and www.longevitywarehouse.com if you are in the United States.

Ron Teeguarden is a leading expert when it comes to herbs; his Dragon Herbs can also be obtained from these sites.

The following descriptions have been adapted from the superfeast and longevitywarehouse websites. Don't forget to go to www.karinaste-phens.com for recipes on tonics, elixirs and juices.

Ginseng

Asian Ginseng is the primary qi tonic of Chinese tonic herbalism. Wild ginseng is an elite Shen tonic, revered by Daoists. Ginseng is one of the most famous and valued herbs used by mankind. *Panax (Asian) Ginseng* is an energy tonic that regulates the human energy system. It helps to regulate and nurture both the central nervous system and the endocrine system.

Ginseng is an adaptogenic herb. It helps a person to adapt to all kinds of stress, and enhances endurance and resilience under stressful conditions. High-quality ginseng tonifies all the systems of the body, but is most specifically tonifying to the spleen and lung functions, the functions that produce Qi in the body.

Wild Ginseng nurtures spiritual power and thus is said to enter the heart meridian. Ginseng contains many active ingredients, but the most important are the saponins called *ginsenosides*. Ginsenosides specifically improve adaptability and are believed to help build muscle and endurance. Therefore Ginseng is very popular with athletes. Asian Ginseng generally has a "warm" energy.

Most high-quality Ginseng is good for men and women alike. Wild and semi-wild Ginseng is generally far superior to the cultivated, commercial varieties. Wild Ginseng possesses qualities that cultivated Ginseng does not, and has been a primary herb used by Daoist adepts. The higher the quality, the more Shen (Spirit) a Ginseng root is said to contain. Beware of cheap Ginseng products, because they are often made from immature roots that have imbalanced chemistry. These cheaper Ginseng products account for Ginseng's unfortunate reputation for increasing tension or for causing headaches, or even high blood pressure. Mature, high-quality Ginseng will not have any side effects.

Reishi mushroom

Reishi mushroom is also known as the "Mushroom of Immortality" and the "Herb of Good Fortune", and is considered by many to be the quintessential tonic herb because of its ability to nurture all three treasures (Jing, Qi, Shen).

Reishi possesses anti-allergenic, anti-inflammatory, anti-viral, anti-bacterial, and antioxidant properties. It has been proven effective in aiding in the treatment of arthritis, and is also an excellent anti-stress herb. When we are holding stress and tension, both physically and mentally, we are compromising our immune system. Our body's ability to fight illness is significantly weakened.

Reishi is known to ease tension, elevate the spirit, and promote peace of mind by transforming negative energy in the body in the same way that the mushroom transforms decayed material in the tree into life-giving nourishment.

Reishi mushroom is a wildcrafted tonic herb for cultivating spiritual energy, modulating immune function, and promoting health, longevity, and peace of mind. It has a legendary status in the Orient because of its ability to profoundly affect so many aspects of our lives in a timely manner.

It is an adaptogenic herb that helps to support and regulate immune function, protect the cardiovascular system, and support and protect the liver. But perhaps its greatest function is that of a Shen tonic. It is unrivalled in its ability to open the heart, calm the spirit, and connect you to your higher self. It enhances wisdom, and supports spiritual evolution and insight.

Chaga

Chaga is unique among medicinal mushrooms and may be one of the most important anti-ageing supplements yet discovered. Like all medicinal mushrooms, Chaga contains the non-linear, complex polysaccharides that give the Chaga extracts potent immune-supporting properties. However, Chaga also has an extremely high ORAC value (antioxidant properties).

Chaga resembles a large piece of burnt charcoal; hence it is sometimes referred to as tinder mushroom. Chaga contains one of the highest amounts of anti-tumour compounds of any of the medicinal mushrooms known, especially in the form of betulinic acid, which is absorbed and concentrates from the birch trees that chaga is commonly found to grow on. Betulin can easily be converted to Betulinic acid which has been shown to possess a wide spectrum of biological activities.

Chaga is also high in vital phytochemicals, nutrients, and free-radical scavenging antioxidants, especially melanin. Melanin is the same compound which is the main pigment in human skin, the retina of the eye, and the pigment-bearing neurons within the brain stem.

Chaga mushroom has marked immuno-stimulatory activity and should be considered by anyone seeking super immunity and longevity.

Ashwagandha: The Indian Ginseng

Ashwagandha is one of the top ten highly beneficial, adaptogenic tonic superherbs, with a strong traditional use in Northern Africa, India, Pakistan, and parts of Asia. It has been used since ancient times for a wide variety of health applications.

In Sanskrit, Ashwagandha means "the smell of a horse". In fact, it's frequently referred to as "Indian Ginseng" because it acts much like Ginseng in effect and effectiveness (botanically, Ginseng and Ashwagandha are unrelated).

Ashwagandha contains many medicinal chemicals, including withanolides (steroidal lactones), alkaloids, choline, fatty acids, amino acids, and a variety of sugars.

He Shou Wu

He Shou Wu is the prepared tuberous root of *Polygonum multiflorum*, a plant that grows in the mountains of central and southern China. It is one of the most important adaptogenic root herbs in Chinese Daoist tonic herbalism.

He Shou Wu is a good source of iron and contains potent antioxidants and antioxidant-potentiating molecules. He Shou Wu supports the body's innate ability to efficiently clear superoxide, the highly reactive free radical, from the body. Free radicals are produced at every moment of our life as part of the living process and our health depends upon our clearing them from our body on a moment-to-moment basis. This support generally comes from foods and herbs humans consume. It is widely believed that the SOD-generating capacity of He Shou Wu is one of the reasons it is considered by many to have "anti-ageing" and "longevity increasing" activity. These actions help maintain healthy physical and mental functions and structures.

He Shou Wu contains zinc, which is an essential trace mineral required by all forms of life. Numerous aspects of cellular metabolism are zinc-dependent. Zinc plays important roles in growth and development, the immune response, neurological function, and reproduction. It is also important to our sexual and reproductive functions.

He Shou Wu has been found to support fundamental immunological functions and to improve adrenal gland functioning.

He Shou Wu is unsurpassed in its ability to provide deep, primordial energy (Jing, essence) to the cells of the body via the kidney system as described in Chinese health philosophy. He Shou Wu supports the human body's "functional reserve".

Schizandra fruit

Schizandra is a wonderful tonic historically consumed by Chinese royalty. It is one of the few herbs that contain all three treasures in abundance. Therefore, all Daoists throughout Chinese history consumed Schizandra.

Schizandra is considered to be a youth-preserving herb and is renowned as a beauty tonic. It has been used for centuries to make the skin soft, moist, and radiant. A powerful tonic to the brain and mind, it is believed in China to improve memory. It is also said to be an excellent and reliable sexual tonic when consumed regularly, helping to produce abundant sexual fluids, increase sexual endurance, and strengthen the whole body.

It is used in many tonic formulations as an "astringent", preventing the leaking of Jing. Schizandra has a wonderful multi-layered flavour when processed properly. The best Schizandra comes from the Chiangbai Mountains of Manchuria (northern China).

Eucommia

Eucommia is one of the primary tonic herbs used throughout Asia for thousands of years to support and mend the skeletal structure, and various tissues throughout the body. It is collected from *Eucommia ulmoides* trees that are more than ten years old.

Eucommia bark is primarily known as a powerful yang Jing tonic, meaning it has the ability to replenish the expansive kidney energy that assists the body in generating strength, stamina, power, and a healthy constitution systemically. Many people use Eucommia because of this to heal from injuries such as broken bones, torn tissue, and ligament damage.

Eucommia also has a strong yin Jing essence, meaning it replenishes the core energy of the body that ensures our baseline health is maintained. Because it provides both yin and yang, it is a great herb for both men and women, and can be used by almost anybody to help support the functions of the skeletal and hormone systems. It is also a wonderful herb to help support healthy sexual functions and libido.

Eucommia is in fact the primary herb in Chinese tonic herbalism for building a strong, sturdy, flexible skeletal structure and to support normal growth.

Astragalus

The root of *Astragalus membranaceus*, a root herb that grows wild in northern China, has been used for over two thousand years to strengthen the immune system and body as a whole. Astragalus is believed by the Oriental people to strengthen muscle and support metabolic functions. One of the most important herbs in the world,

Astragalus has been recognised as a superb and potent tonic by modern researchers.

Astragalus is said to have an effect on the "surface" of the body; that is, it is used to tonify the "Protective Q", known as Wei Qi in Chinese. This Protective Qi is a special kind of energy which circulates just under the skin and in the muscle. Protective Qi is a yang energy. Protective Qi circulates in the subcutaneous tissues providing suppleness to the flesh and adaptive energy to the skin. This function is essential to life. Wei Qi is the energy of the skin and immune system, in harmony, that responds to changes in the environment.

Rehmannia

Rehmannia is one of the most important Chinese herbs for supporting the kidneys and adrenal glands, and is even thought to support the pituitary gland. Rehmannia also appears to combat adrenal suppression caused by steroid hormones and has a similar tonic effect on the adrenal cortex as liquorice tonic effect on the adrenal cortex as liquorice. Thought to be powerfully immuno-supportive, Rehmannia is also used to help promote a healthy inflammation response, along with herbs such as bupleurum. It is also known to support libido, joint health, respiratory health, and healthful ageing.

CHAPTER 10

Building A Stress Defence Shield

What is it in your life that is causing you the most stress right at this very moment? Is it the lack of finances, struggling to pay the bills on time, or the ever-increasing debt? Is it your job that you go to five days a week and every day your soul dies a little bit more because you can't stand the environment, or your boss, or that colleague who makes your life hell?

Is it a health issue, which prevents you from living life to the full? Or the diagnosis of a life-threatening disease for you or someone you love?

Whatever the cause, think about how it makes you feel. What emotions do you experience on a daily basis? How do you feel in your body when you think about it? What sort of person are you becoming because of it?

Imagine if we could have a superhero power which is the ability to deflect stress? How would this change your life? What if that situation that causes you the most stress didn't have the same effect on you because you had built a shield around yourself which was diminishing its effect? Would you laugh more, love more, have the courage to change jobs, or go into business for yourself? Would you stop resisting that diagnosis and start believing in miracles?

Well, I am here to tell you that anyone can have this superpower. There is such a thing as a stress defence shield and it has changed my life more than I can say.

When I was completing David Wolfe's Raw Nutrition certification I learned that we have access to a stress defence shield, which literally drives the stress off us. Whoa, how come I didn't know this before? This little pearl sent me into an excitable little sweat, because if I could learn how to build a defence shield around me that would be like having super powers.

After a lot of research and investigating I learnt exactly what a stress defence shield is and how we can all have this super power.

What I have come to realise is that we can build this shield using three key areas. First of all we can physically eat the right foods in order to produce the right hormones and neurotransmitters, which will ignite our shield. We can also strengthen it spiritually by meditating and using affirmations. Thirdly, we can build our stress defence shield energetically by practising a few simple techniques.

I have kept the following information simple. I have tried to cut out technical jargon and make it as practical as possible. For the purpose of this book, my aim is to show you the basics and not overwhelm you. I have been my own crash test dummy. I have done the research, I have studied with the gurus like David Wolfe, Donna Eden and Louise Hay, and I have the proof by the healing that has occurred in my life. As with anything, there is no one-size-fits-all, and so my aim is to show you how you can become so in tune with your body that it will tell you exactly what you need in order to heal.

This is what happens: we eliminate or drastically reduce the cause of inflammation, dis-ease and stress in our bodies, and then it has the space to start to restore itself back to its natural state. During this process our intuition heightens; we become far more sensitive to what is making us ill. As we continue to restore we then have a chance to rebuild and regain what was depleted.

By concentrating on developing a defence field for stress we can drastically reduce the chance of stress ever affecting us to the degree where we have become burnt out, stressed out, maxed out, and, you got it, checked out again.

I have tried each and every one of the techniques and processes I am about to share with you. You do not need to do them all, just do what feels right for you in this moment. Then over time you may be directed to add or try another one. The point is not to add more things on your "to do" list, so keep it simple. Give yourself the gift of committing to even just one new thing for a month and then see how you feel. If you feel the change keep doing it.

For me, I wanted the best darn shield I could have for my super-power. Over time it became more powerful, as it strengthened each day I drank my superhero smoothie, or committed to the energy work. The same can happen to you as well, I guarantee it.

Building our stress defence shield physically

So let's look at building our stress defence shield physically first. Essentially it is a build-up of three neurotransmitters which work together to create a shield which drives stress off us.

The first is serotonin, which is our feel-good hormone. The greater the level of serotonin, the more capable we are of pushing the stress out of our bodies.

The second is the phenethylamines that include hormones and neurotransmitters such as adrenaline and noradrenaline. When our adrenal glands, pituitary, and hypothalamus are working efficiently and producing these substances, we are more likely to ward off stress.

The third neurotransmitter is dopamine, allowing us to focus and work. Researchers are looking at high levels of dopamine actually keeping us younger because it is a human growth hormone.

We can actually build up our stress defence shield by ingesting substances every day which produce these substances, and it is relatively easy to do.

Firstly, if we remove electromagnetic pollution fields and get away from the stresses of life as often as we can, our defence shield will certainly come up because we are able to build up our level of dopamine.

This is because we are not having the stimulants which deplete this; we are calming our whole nervous system. However, given that we live in polluted cities and travel and live the lifestyles that we do, it can take more effort to stay clean, green, and conscious. Simply concentrating on adding a couple of certain types of food in our diet will go towards increasing our defence shield.

With serotonin we have to have foods which contain tryptophan, or we take supplements. Tryptophan is found in all high-protein foods, and I believe the best source is from superfoods. A great resource to have is David Wolfe's book *Superfoods: The Food and Medicine of the Future*; it has all the research and information on this type of nutrition.

Foods such as goji berries, maca, spirulina, marine phytoplankton, chlorella, and bee pollen are all classed as superfoods and excellent sources of tryptophan. By adding these foods into our diet we start to feel good. That's because they are producing neurotransmitters. We are finally loading our system with all the good stuff and it is letting us know that it is feeling really good inside.

In his online course, "The Ultimate Raw Nutrition Course", David states that he believes serotonin is influenced by the sun; the more sunlight we get on our skin the more serotonin we produce. We produce vitamin D3 when we have sunlight on our skin and so when we are in places which do not get a lot of sun, taking a vitamin D3 supplement can be extremely beneficial.

Now, let's move onto phenethylamines. Cacao is very rich in these and also very rich in tryptophan. It also contains some dopamine. Blue-green algae also includes phenethylamines and I add both of these into my morning superhero smoothie, which I have included the recipe of in this chapter.

When we have a hit of stimulants such as cigarettes or coffee day after day, it wipes out our dopamine. It is the hormone related to going out and relating to the world. One of the most powerful precursors to dopamine is a bean called Mucuna; it contains L-dopa and is a great Jing herb.

Another great source is deer antler but I recommend you do your research and make sure you buy it from a reputable farmer who practises humane standards for its deer. Collecting the antler should not hurt the deer as the antler grows back over time.

So now we have gathered a few types of sources for serotonin, phenethylamines, and dopamine, we need to add part two of building our stress defence shield which is what David Wolfe describes as decoupling stress from our immune system.

We have to get our immune system up so that it is not tapping into our stress. There are a number of substances which help to do this which are really easy to add to any diet. I just throw them in my morning smoothie and I don't even think about it for the rest of the day.

Vitamin C botanicals like camu camu berry, powdered rosehips, or amla berry can help to really amp up the immune system. Combine this with the power of medicinal mushrooms and the phycocyanin contained in blue-green algae and we now have an immune system that is able to function and produce weapons.

I must admit I was a bit overwhelmed when I first started researching all of the foods which contain the substances needed for building a defence shield. I thought to myself, *bloody hell, how am I going to add all of this to my diet?* But over time and as my budget allowed I was able to stock up on most of what I needed. Then I just decided to add it all to my green smoothie I was making every morning anyway.

So here is the recipe for my superhero smoothie. You can add all of the ingredients or just some. Trust me, a few is better than none and then adjust the measurements to your own little taste buds' liking.

Superhero green smoothie

Coconut water
1 tsp maca powder
1 tsp wheat grass powder
A few goji berries
1 tsp Pepitas
1 tsp Sunflower Seeds

1 tsp Hemp seeds
Blue-green algae
1 tsp Udo's Oil
1 tsp spirulina
1 tsp MSM
1 tbs cacao
1 handful of kale or spinach
1/3 cup of organic blueberries

Blend all ingredients in a high-powered blender and enjoy. I also make a stress defence shield tea which knocks your little cotton socks off. You can find the recipe at www.karinastephens.com/pog-gifts

Building our stress defence shield energetically

Have you ever spent time with someone and when you walk away you feel totally drained? If you have, then you have just been slimed, my dear. Some well-meaning person has just drained you of your energy and now you feel like crap.

A good healer and therapist knows how to shield themselves from taking on other people's energy. There are a number of ways in which you can do this but I found the best way for me was to do a simple little energy technique called the Celtic weave. I learnt this from Donna Eden who is an amazing energy healer. I recommend checking out her website if you really want to learn more about energy medicine at http://innersource.net/em/

The Celtic weave strengthens the energy field around you and protects you from harmful energies in the environment. Performing this technique every day and whenever you know you are going to be around a lot of people will create a stress defence shield around you and help to protect you.

Celtic weave technique

Begin by allowing a nice deep breath and then rub your hands together really fast so you begin to feel them heat up.

Shake off your hands and then hold your palms close to your ears.

Now inhale bringing your elbows together in front of you, exhale crossing your arms, then swing out wide.

Cross and swing again, bend forward, and repeat crossing arms over your upper legs, then ankles.

Turn palms forward, scoop up the energy, slowly stand, and pour that energy all over the body.

I have added a short video on my website to help demonstrate the Celtic weave; just go to www.karinastephens.com/pog-gifts for all your resources.

Building our stress defence shield spiritually

Affirmations are powerful tools in creating and transforming our lives. I use affirmations all the time when I am working on healing or creating something new and extraordinary.

When I was healing from adrenal fatigue and wanting to build up my stress defence shield, this was the affirmation I created for myself. I wrote it on Post-its and stuck it up all over my home. You can easily tailor it to suit you personally or just use mine.

Every day in every way I trust that I am strengthening my stress defence shield, and that it is protecting me from negative and harmful energies. I am safe and I am loved.

Every day in every way I am becoming more and more resilient to what used to stress me out. Struggle and strain are now making way for ease and joy. I am perfect just as I am.

As you say this affirmation as often as you can throughout the day, visualise yourself surrounded by a shield of luminous white light. This light is protecting you, and as you continue to practise the techniques I have just shared with you, it grows stronger and stronger each day.

So now that you are becoming a superhero with a mighty stress defence shield, you will begin to notice that your body is becoming far more resilient to disease because you are strengthening your immune system with all those wonderful superfoods.

You will become aware that you have more energy left over at the end of the day because it hasn't been zapped by people you have come in contact with.

And you will start to realise that your negative self-talk is becoming quieter and softer. Emotionally you feel stronger and more grounded.

The secret is in the word "consistency". The more committed you are to these practices and the other techniques in this book, the faster you will feel yourself travelling at the Pace of Grace. Slowly over time your kryptonite will no longer immobilise you because you've let go of the stress, struggle, and fatigue of life. You have slowed down enough to hear the sweet whisper of the StressLess sage guiding you in your selah moments. You are now practising unapologetic self-love and you are removing the blocks to ease, joy, and abundance.

That, my friend, is a pretty amazing superpower to have, don't you think?

CHAPTER 11

Doing Less Physically And More Energetically

I recently heard an interview with Anthony William who is a medical medium. He stated that 85% of Americans have some sort of adrenal fatigue, ranging from mild to severe. I guess the same can be said for anyone living in the Western world. That's a lot of people dragging their feet around, just trying to make it through the day.

We get up tired; we operate on autopilot all day. We do the bare minimum just to get by. We are reacting to the slightest things emotionally. There is a numbness which we have spun around ourselves like a cocoon in order to protect ourselves from being overstimulated.

We think that going on a holiday will fix us but it won't. It just temporarily helps us to forget. We drink more coffee and ingest other stimulants in order to get us going and then we reach for the alcohol or the mind-numbing television at night to bring us down.

It's like life is doing us rather than we are doing life. Eventually we can't take it anymore: the stress, the struggle and the strain become too much so our little bodies will force us to slow down or completely stop. I got adrenal fatigue. Others get fibromyalgia, chronic fatigue, have a bad accident or some other illness manifests into their life.

If this has happened to you then ask yourself the question, "What is it I need to know?"

I am a qualified facilitator in Heal your Life, the program created by Louise Hay. In her book with the same name, Louise states that every physical symptom has an emotional cause. This little book has changed countless lives around the world and if you haven't read it I suggest you go out and buy a copy today.

When I asked myself that question, "What is it I need to know?," the answer that came back was not one I expected. The answer I received said, "You need to do less physically and more energetically."

Interesting—in the past no matter how much I tried to change, to work harder, no matter how many hours I put in at work or at the gym, I could never truly tap into the Pace of Grace and experience life being one of effortless ease and flow. My experience was that if I took my hands off the wheel of life, I would be in the car with Thelma and Louise going right on over the cliff.

If I was truly honest after 44 years, this way of living just ended up with me in bed for most of the day and the rest of the day with my legs up the wall in a restorative yoga pose.

So I pondered on what it meant to do less physically and more energetically. Whilst my body rested in gentle yoga poses and slept more than a baby the answers started to awaken me.

I started to get it: we are so busy running around practising the art of being busy that all we have achieved is a state of being bloody tired. If we were to take some time to look at our emotions, energetic bodies and spiritual life then maybe we could tap into the Pace of Grace and experience a life of effortless ease and flow.

When I was first diagnosed with adrenal fatigue my initial reaction was that I had to make physical changes in order for me to cure myself. Whilst this was somewhat true, the most profound changes occurred when I started to work with my energy.

Several years before I had started to develop severe allergies. I had test after test and they seemed to indicate I was allergic to just about everything. These allergies seemed to strip me of my energy and if anyone who suffers from them knows, there is a fog and a constant irritation that won't leave.

As well as the allergies I was starting to have an increased sensitivity to noise, light and large crowds. This heightened over the years to the point where I would avoid any event where a large number of people would be, because it would just exhaust me.

Each time I went to the shopping centre I would feel like I was having this concrete contraction in my soul. What used to be fun was now draining my energy severely.

I tried exercising more in order to lose the 10 kilograms of weight I had put on. I changed my diet, limited the times I shopped, but nothing was working. I was becoming sensitive and it pissed me off. I thought I was becoming weak.

During my sabbatical of wellness I had a very enlightened reading with my astrologist who kindly pointed out, "Karina, you're sensitive."

No shit!

But she went on to inform me that my sensitivity is like an orchid. She said, "We don't plant you in the front garden with the other flowers, you go in the hot house."

She made me realise my 'orchidness' was a gift and I was abusing it. So I started to treat it like one. I read books on being sensitive; I listened to audio files and watched videos.

I started to see my energy as just as important as my physical health. As blood pumps through our veins, energy courses through our chakras and meridians. If these are blocked with stress, we don't function fully.

So I started to do all kinds of things that made my husband look at me with some major WTF faces but he eventually came around. I started saging the house with white sage in order to neutralise the energy. I dove into the world of energy medicine and learnt how to clear energy blocks therefore increasing my life force. I upped my meditation practice and learnt all about angels and spirit guides.

All of these tools and practices assisted me in clearing my allergies and increasing my energy. It was working on my energy that helped me shift into the Pace of Grace.

Once I had cleared the stress blocks energetically it felt like every other area was able to open up to a deeper level of healing. As I cleared stress blocks from my emotional and physical body, I felt the years of weariness, exhaustion and fatigue float away. With each release I was able to step into a higher vibration of being. I wasn't being held back by negative thoughts and destructive patterns of behaviour.

Slowly, I realised I didn't need that nap in the afternoon; I actually woke up feeling like I got eight hours' sleep. I didn't have to drag my butt around all day just trying to get through everything that needed to get done. My butt was high off the ground and happy to be there.

There were obviously good days and not-so-good days but that was what I needed in order for me to learn how my energy worked. On the not-so-great days, I rested and didn't feel guilty. I nourished my body with awesome live foods. I practised my energy medicine techniques. On the good days I was able to be more physical; I went for a walk or did a yoga class. I was able to sit down at the computer and work.

Once I thought that the only way to reach my dreams, to achieve anything in life and to get ahead was to work hard, do my goal setting and vision boards with ferocious determination, keep up with the pace of life and live in the rat race.

Now I know this way just gets you burnt out. I can still reach my dreams; I can achieve anything I want in life. I can live in affluence and experience abundance every day and do it all with ease and joy.

We think to lose those extra kilos we need to run our butts into the road and push through the exhaustion. Get our bodies into the gym every day without fail and eat whatever the latest fad diet is.

Can I just tell you now that if you are burnt out, stressed out, maxed out or checked out this way of trying to lose weight will only make you fatter. In chapter 12, I explain why this is but for now just know that you have my permission to put the gym bag away for a while and rest.

Your body needs rest in order to repair and the more you continue to slam it up against the weights bench the more you will produce the hormones which continue to put weight on.

We talked in chapter 7 about the intuitive chakra and how opening and clearing this chakra can increase our intuition. Performing a complete chakra cleanse is another technique which opens up our seven chakras allowing direct flow to each and every area of our energy system. Our chakras are all connected so if we are blocked in one particular chakra, energy is unable to reach our higher chakras.

I have a simple meditation I perform whenever I feel I need to do a more involved clearing which I have included for you below. You can also obtain the MP3 from http://www.karinastephens.com/pog-gifts

Chakra Meditation Clearing

Close your eyes and turn your vision inwards. Become aware of your body, as you breathe deeply. Feel your body sink deeper into relaxation; with every breath feel your muscles soften. With every exhale, feel your whole body slow down.

The exhalation is our brake; it's a chance to unwind, soften, and be still.

Imagine a warm, glowing white light in the centre of your body; this light is like a pilot light, gently flickering. Now when you are ready see this light ignited and filling your entire body and aura with a luminous glow.

This feels warm and healing. Your whole body is now soft and illuminated with this soft white healing light.

Now bring your attention to the base of your spine. See or feel a red glowing light of physical energy spinning like a fan. This is your root chakra, your balance starts here. Spend some time picturing a ball of ruby red light glowing strongly at the base of your spine and reproductive region. See if you can notice any dark spots, discolourations, or distortions. If you do notice this, allow your healing white light to dissolve all darkness until all you see is a perfect circle of spinning ruby red light.

Say to yourself:

"I trust that I am safe and divinely guided and protected", "I trust in myself", "I trust life supports me in fulfilling my purpose". Now allow an inhalation of breath followed by a loud exhale with a sigh.

Next, bring your attention to about three inches below your belly button and see or feel a ball of spinning orange energy. This is your sacral chakra, the area for socialising, intimacy, sensuality, and freedom.

Scan this area for any dark spots, discolourations, or distortions. If you do notice them, allow your healing white light to dissolve all darkness until all you see is a perfect circle of spinning orange light. Say to yourself:

"I trust my own creativity", "I trust that it is safe to allow pleasure, sweetness and sensuality into my life", "I trust my deepest insights".

Now allow a vibrational breath by inhaling followed by a loud exhale and sigh.

Now rest your attention on the area below your rib cage. See or feel a bright yellow colour like a small sun. This is your solar plexus chakra, the area associated with personal will, mental clarity, self-esteem, and the ability to take action.

Scan this area for any dark spots, discolourations, or distortions. If you do notice them, allow your healing white light to dissolve all darkness until all you see is a perfect circle of spinning yellow light. Say to yourself:

"I trust that I am enough", "I trust that I am worthy of my own self-love", "I trust that I have the power within me to follow my purpose".

Next, allow a vibrational breath by inhaling followed by a loud exhalation sigh.

Now we come up to the centre of our chest, our heart chakra; see or feel a beautiful emerald green light shining from your heart chakra. This chakra is associated with your ability to love and accept love, your appreciation and gratitude for life. If you see or feel any darkness then dissolve this by allowing your beautiful healing white light to illuminate the darkness. Say to yourself:

"I trust in love", "I trust that all my mistakes happened so that I can learn to forgive myself", " I trust in and follow the path of my heart".

Now allow a vibrational breath.

Coming up to our neck and our throat chakra we see or feel a ball of light blue spinning energy. This chakra is associated with speaking your truth. If you see or feel any darkness then dissolve this by allowing your beautiful healing white light to illuminate the darkness. Say to yourself:

"I trust that it is safe to speak my truth today", "I trust that old patterns which have been blocking me in the past are now removed", "I trust in the power of my own voice". Now allow a vibrational breath.

Next we move up to the area located between our eyes. This is known as our third eye chakra, the area associated with intuition, imagination, mental clarity, clairvoyance, and the ability to see life clearly.

See or feel a dark blue colour with the occasional flashes of purple or white; scan this area for any dark spots, discolourations, or distortions. If you do notice them, allow your healing white light to dissolve all darkness until all you see is a perfect circle of spinning dark blue light by saying:

"I trust that it is now safe to open myself to intuition and deepest knowing", "I trust that it is now safe to be open to new ideas, people and opportunities", "I trust that whatever comes to me is for my greatest joy and highest good".

Take a deep breath and exhale with a loud sigh.

Now bring your attention to the top of your head, the area associated with your crown chakra. See or feel a vibrant purple colour spinning like a fan. This is the area associated with wisdom, spiritual awareness, and awakening. Scan this area for any dark spots, discolourations, or distortions. If you do notice them, allow your healing white light to dissolve all darkness until all you see is a perfect circle of spinning purple light. Say to yourself:

"I trust in the oneness of life", "I trust that I am divinely protected and guided", "I trust that it is now safe to be responsible for the quality of life I enjoy".

Allow a vibrational breath.

Finally, take the time to focus on the interaction of your chakras; picture all of them together, sharing, harmonising, and feeding ideas and power to each other. Continue to breathe easily, basking in the love and healing energy, and then when you are ready gently open your eyes, coming back to this moment in time.

Taking the stress out of finding your lover for life

Another example where doing less physically and more energetically can really work is if you are trying to find your lover for life. It can be very stressful when you desire a romantic partner, someone to share your life with. A lot of us can get into that desperate energy when we feel like it is taking forever to find the right one.

For ten years I was single and searching for THE ONE. I did all the things single girls do: went to all the right places, signed up on all the right online dating sites. It wasn't until I stopped doing all the physical stuff and started looking deeper that I found him.

The Merriam-Webster online dictionary describes the word "surrender" as: v: *to give oneself up into the power of another*. We don't like to relinquish control of our lives to someone else, do we? I know that I loved to be in control of my life because then I had a perceived sense of power. To give that power to someone else takes faith—faith that this someone will look after you and do right by you. Faith is the substance of things unseen.

This law was the hardest for me to learn because I resisted it for so long. How can I trust God to find me the right partner when God is so busy saving the world, right? Wrong! Oh me of little faith. Ian couldn't be more perfect for me than if I had created him myself. Actually, if I had created him myself then I wouldn't have put in all the little things about him that so brilliantly bring out the character flaws in me.

I literally had to come to a place of surrender and give up the struggle and the search in order to let go and let God. I was so busy going about my business of getting out of club "singledom" that I hadn't given God any room to move. When I say "give up" I don't mean give up the desire, I mean give up the struggle and the fear that covet the desire. Get to the place in your heart where you truly believe that you will be okay if you never have a partner. That life will still be full and blessed and abundant in other ways. You will still have a wonderful life. When you do this you allow the energy of life to flow freely again.

You've heard the expression "you'll find love when you're not looking". Sometimes when you give the very thing you want the most back to your creator then He will give it back in a way that you could never have dreamed of, even more special and out of this world.

I remember vividly the moment I presented my desire for a life partner to God. I was in my little apartment one night. I had cooked a beautiful dinner, set the table with my best dinner set, lit the candles, and had Michael Bublé serenading me in the background.

As I looked into the most loving brown eyes I had ever known, the eyes of my little dog, I knew in my heart that I had to die to my dream in order for me to be the best me that I could be. Because whilst I was living in this state of struggle and fear, I would never know the freedom that came from releasing this state. I would never know the magic of "being content in the moment" and I would never know the peace that comes from living with faith.

That night, I got down on my knees, I put my little dream man in a box and wrapped him up with gold paper and a bright red ribbon, and I presented him to my God as a gift. I prayed, "God, I'm giving my dream to you and if one day you should choose to gift it back to me then I will be a very, very happy girl but if you don't then I promise to live my life being the best me that I can be."

God gave my gift to Him back to me but it was way different than the one I'd given Him. I gave Him a desired partner and He gave me back a Lover for Life. I gave Him the dream of an ordinary man and He gave me back an extraordinary man of God. I gave Him the hope of a good marriage and He gave me the promise of eternal love. I gave Him my heart and He gave me my TRUE destiny.

If you are experiencing a lot of struggle and strain in any area of your life right now, and you seem to be pushing jelly up a hill because nothing is changing, then listen up.

Have you ever asked yourself how come this always happens to you? Have you ever thought that you must have done something wrong in a previous life because you sure do have a shitload of bad luck in this one? Muttered the words, "just my luck" more than once?

These words create a certain vibration, one that has a lower frequency. When we are tuned into this vibration we attract all the things we don't want because that is where our focus is.

I was so in tune to the frequency of lack, struggle, and stress that it was number one on my playlist. Oh, there were times when I changed the channel and wow, I just received a cheque for one thousand dollars in the mail. But I couldn't sustain the vibration. My old conditioning led me straight back to what I knew best.

It wasn't until I addressed the stress blocks, which were literally strangling my energy and holding my emotions captive, that I was able to break free of the energy of stress, struggle, and lack. Many, many selah moments later I can now say that those days are well behind me.

And this will be the same for you as well. When you begin to work with your mindset, your emotions, and your energetic body, life will start to unravel. As you begin to slow down the energy around you shifts. Where once there was an erratic, frantic, and chaotic feeling, it is replaced with a calmer and softer energy.

It is in this energy where your body starts to restore itself. Struggle dissolves into ease, stress disappears into joy, and lack transcends into abundance.

CHAPTER 12

Rest And Restoration

I think we are all up to date by now with the benefit that fitness has on our lives. We understand the effect which exercise has on our body. We know that we need to get huffy puffy in order to have a strong heart and cardiovascular system. We have heard that in order to lose weight we need to move our butts and sweat baby sweat.

Well, what if I was to tell you that if you are burnt out, stressed out, maxed out, and checked out, then I don't want you doing any of that? Yep, you have my permission not to jog, to ditch the Zumba class, and boohoo the treadmill. Your body doesn't need any more stress; it needs to rest for a while and this chapter is where you get to slow down and try a little Savasana.

During the first eight years of my marriage I put on ten kilos. That's more than a kilo a year and, no, I am not blaming my gorgeous husband. It was also the period that I moved into my forties, where my nervous system said enough to my previous lifestyle and began to rebel, and where life persuaded me to go slower than I've ever gone, in order to go deeper than I've ever been.

I am only five feet four inches tall, so ten extra kilograms on my small frame was a lot, and if you have ever been overweight you can understand that with the excess weight often comes critical feelings of self-loathing and judgment. I would look in the mirror and see only my faults: my big belly and the folds over my bra strap. I knew I wasn't the best version of myself physically and this made me sad.

Like most people I tried to lose the weight; I focused on it a lot. I changed my diet lots of times, I ramped up the cardio, increased the sit-ups, yet all I could manage was to yo-yo up and down. This pressure I put on myself to lose the weight was stressing me out and then my body went into burnout and I couldn't even lift my head off the pillow, let alone do a sit-up.

For the first four months of my healing I couldn't even go for an exercise walk and this pissed me off so much. I thought I needed to be active in order to heal but what I really needed was rest and recovery. I had to lose the guilt associated with being inactive. I thought I was being lazy but what I was actually doing was conscious restoration. Me actually listening to my body when I was overcome with fatigue and going to lie down was more beneficial for me than going for an exercise walk. As soon as I made peace with this, the angst went away. The moment I surrendered into the reality of what was for the moment, my body softened. The struggle and strain completely dissolved and I was able to enjoy the activity of being inactive.

After about three months, I felt rested enough to try restorative yoga. This is a very gentle supported yoga, especially designed to support the nervous system. This turned out to be so beneficial in my healing that I continue the practice today.

Within four months, I started to feel my energy was strong enough to go for short walks. I started to walk about fifteen minutes a day at a really gentle pace and gradually I was able to build this up to a forty-five-minute walk three to four times a week. There were days where I knew I should rest and not exercise and when I listened to this whisper and did what I was told, I would usually have restored my energy enough to go out the next day. If I ignored it and pushed through and went for that darned walk anyway, it would wipe me out for the week.

You get good at paying attention to your body; you start to feel the amount of energy you have in your system. When you begin your day with presence and awareness it will reveal all this information to you.

It wasn't until about twelve months into my healing when I knew that I could go the next level. I had wanted to do a more physical yoga for a few months yet every time I felt into if it was the right time, I always got a no. Now twelve months was not my time frame, I can tell you that; I expected to be up and about and back to the gym within six, but having expectations on time when it comes to your healing can only lead to suffering. I soon learnt I had to let that go and just continue being led and guided, all the while trusting that everything was as it should be.

I started hot yoga because I knew it would help with my detoxification as well as provide all the other benefits which yoga has on the body. I absolutely loved it and I could feel my body growing stronger each day.

What happened as I took the focus off my weight and onto my healing was that the weight started to release; it was effortless, I wasn't even trying. It is incredibly hard to lose weight when your body is acidic and as I adopted a very alkaline lifestyle, my body was able to release the acidity and regain homeostasis. As of today I weigh the same as I did fifteen years ago. Since adopting the StressLess nutrition plan, I now have my energy back and can enjoy high-cardio activities again because my body is strong enough to deal with the stress. It's a good stress, not the chronic bad stress that we focus on in this book. I never count calories, or look at the scales, or worry about what I eat because I know that what I eat is healthy and nutritious, and the most powerful foods on the planet.

I share my journey with you because I know a lot of people who are suffering from fatigue and feel that they need to push through and do some hard-core exercise in order to be healthy. Running actually raises cortisol levels and when you are trying to decrease cortisol this is not a good thing to do. When their body gives out on them they experience guilt and frustration. We need to be kinder to ourselves, we need to know that if we have tapped out our adrenals or compromised our systems in any way, they don't need to be put under extra pressure, they need to be supported and nourished.

Then when we have aligned ourselves back with our natural state, we can move into a more active exercise program. Even if you are not burnt out, you still need to add a rest and restore component to your day. We want to be the best we can be, achieve our goals, live our dreams, and be there for our loved ones: this is all a natural part of being a healthy, vibrant, alive human being. But unless we include rest and restoration into the picture, we will eventually burn out.

By rest and restoration I am not talking about sitting on the couch doing nothing: it is conscious downtime designed to restore your nervous system and bring you into the para-sympathetic nervous system, which is your rest and digest state.

Below are my favourite activities to help you achieve this and by committing even fifteen minutes a day you will be miles ahead of the game. Normally I will include a twenty-minute meditation with a thirty-minute activity first thing in the morning and this sets me up for the day. I love variety so I might do a walk one day, a yoga session the next, and qigong on the third day. How you structure your rest and restoration time is up to you; the main thing is to do what you love and value this time as an important part of your StressLess lifestyle.

Restoration activities

Meditation
Meditation actually aligns the nervous system, takes you out of the fight-or-flight response, and calms down your entire internal organs and systems. With so many benefits it is a wonder everyone doesn't do it. If you want to live a StressLess lifestyle then, sweetie, you're going to have to commit to this beautiful practice on a consistent basis and when you do I promise you life will never be the same again.

I started off with five minutes a day listening to different guided meditations and built that up to twenty minutes twice a day. I am not saying you have to do this but I'm sure that in the end you'll want to. The trick is to not beat yourself up; you can't get it wrong, it's a win win. At the beginning of your practice be as gentle with yourself as you would a new baby learning to walk. Love yourself through this and as you do life will love you back ten-fold.

The aim is to not stop your thoughts but to not be engaged with them. When you notice them, and you will, that's a certainty, just imagine them float down the river and then go back to your breath or your mantra. There are so many meditation styles and practices around that you are certain to find the one which suits your personality. Try them all and have fun with the process; treat it as a priority and you will soon be living life at the Pace of Grace.

Restorative yoga

Restorative yoga consists of poses, pranayama, breath awareness exercises, and meditation. The para-sympathetic nervous system is activated during restorative yoga. To do this props are used to firstly support the body so no strain or striving occurs. Specific breath and mind awareness is applied before and during the pose. If you Google gentle yoga or restorative yoga you will find a multitude of videos. I love Gaia TV as it has some wonderful yoga sessions, and because I subscribe I get to experience a huge array of instructors and trainers and find the ones I like best. You may even find a local class close to where you live and do a series of sessions.

Sleep

I know that this may sound like a "well, duhhhh" but most of us do not sleep enough. Most of us need to be getting eight to ten hours of sleep when we are burnt out in order for our bodies to be able to heal and restore balance. Even when we are operating at our peak performance we still need seven to eight hours of good, solid sleep, otherwise we start the day operating like a V8 car running on only four cylinders. Sleep energises and restores us back to peak performance, so don't dismiss it.

If you are someone who can operate at your highest capacity on only 4-5 hours sleep, then you go you good thing. Just a disclaimer, there is a difference between only needing 5 hours sleep and only getting 5 hours sleep. We just have to be honest with ourselves here and tune into our body.

Also, it's best to be in bed and asleep between nine p.m. and ten-thirty p.m. before the next dump of adrenaline hits around eleven p.m.

Also don't dismiss the benefit of a power nap. Having a midday si-esta can improve mood, alertness, and performance.

Walking

Walking in nature is one of the most restorative activities you can partake in. Walking helps burn off and reduce the adrenaline and nora-drenaline that has been released in your bloodstream via the stress re-sponse. A thirty-minute walk can significantly reduce your stress, improve your mood and get you back into the Pace of Grace.

A great practice whilst walking is to think about all the things you are grateful for in your life. Focusing on the hip area will put you back into your power centre, grounding you. Visualising light coming from your heart chakra out into the world will connect you with mother earth.

Stretching

In his book, *The Genius Of Flexibility: The Smart Way to Stretch and Strengthen your Body*, Robert Cooley says, "Unbelievable spiritual changes result from developing greater flexibility. Becoming more flexible connects you with positive life changes while it disconnects you from objectionable parts of your life. Changes in awareness and modifications in perspective become daily occurrences. You can di-rectly experience the wonderful connection between your body and your life from stretching. You find yourself making better choices, showing greater integrity, and enjoying doing the things that are good for you. You begin to live more and suffer less, experiencing everything about energy and spirit, living timelessly."

I believe this makes total sense: by stretching for twenty minutes a day we reconnect to our bodies; we breathe into the muscles, tendons and ligaments. We begin to release the tension and contraction from within, and restore balance and harmony into our physicality.

CHAPTER 13

You Are One Thought Away From Peace

Dr Wayne Dyer said that we are always just one thought away from peace. Finding that thought in a moment of frustration, anger, or suffering is the miracle. A course in miracles says that we do not know how to deal with the situation serenely because of our thoughts about what happened.

It is not the event; it is how we respond to the event that matters. Our response determines the amount of stress, struggle, and suffering that we will experience. Our response is also a great indicator of the gap to our enlightenment.

As I write this book I got to see that gap in all its glory, thanks to a little company, which will remain nameless. Without going into too much of the gory details, my call to customer service took over two hours, which led me no closer to fixing my problem.

It did, however, lead me to tears over the phone, complete adrenal exhaustion, and being fried for the rest of the day. In my review of how I could have handled it better or differently, I realised it was my thoughts that these people are not helping me, they are just passing me from department to department, they do not know what they are doing, they do not want to help me, and my best one, they are complete morons.

Have you ever been in a situation with a customer service company where "service" is a word added in to elicit humour? For starters, you are on hold for what seems like an eternity, then you get the rep from hell who is determined to do everything in their power not to give you what you need. What starts off as a polite request soon escalates into a scene from the Dr Phil show, and then to top it off you get cut off and you know it was so not an accident.

I have been on both ends of the phone, having worked in a call centre, so I can speak from both sides here. It is not pretty, and there is always a better way to handle things if we take the emotion out of it.

Presence offers the greatest ability to be aware of what you are thinking in any given moment. Awareness offers the greatest ability to change those thoughts.

Firstly, I wasn't present in that conversation with the service representatives from this company. I was in the future seeing all the possibilities of what could happen if they didn't fix my problem. Secondly, I wasn't aware I was thinking all the thoughts that were causing me to stress out; I was so caught up in the story, I couldn't see the thoughts that were creating the story.

If I had have been present, in the now moment, I could have seen it wasn't the end of the world. No one is going to die; it is not the end of the world if they can't fix my problem, it will just take some creative thinking and extra effort to find a way around. Sure, it is annoying but it is not worth compromising my health for.

If I had been aware of my thoughts, I would have realised they were all fear-based thoughts, they were not coming from a place of love. They were also not the truth; I didn't know for sure that they did not want to help me. I could not be 100 percent positive that they were actual morons. If it is not the truth then it is not real; anything that comes from fear is not real.

Now, I can hear you saying, "Well, that's all fine, Karina, but it's a bit harder to be present and aware in the actual moment, all the time." Fair call, my friend, and that is why our goal should be not to achieve perfection but to have less and less of the out-of-control, devil possessed moments. And how we achieve this is through adopting and practising meditation, prayer, and self-actualisation.

By adopting a consistent spiritual practice over time we don't get triggered as easily. What used to bring us to anger is now no longer an issue. We are grounding ourselves in what A Course in Miracles describes as the vertical realm, which is our relationship with the divine. The horizontal realm is the realm of the mortal and the way to be empowered in the mortal realm is to be aligned with vertical realm.

When our spiritual lives are aligned the peaceful thoughts are effortless. It is easier to reach for a peaceful thought because they vibrate at a higher frequency. When we maintain a spiritual practice we raise our vibration up to meet these thoughts. When negative thoughts enter our mind we can be aware without being engaged. We can acknowledge the thought as separate from ourselves and in doing so maintain a peaceful response to a situation, which could otherwise stress us out.

Another way to locate that beautiful thought which would bring you peace is to reach for a better healing feeling. What do I mean by that?

Our emotions can be measured by how good we feel when we feel a particular feeling. There are a number of emotional scales on the internet which rate each emotion from highest to lowest, the lowest being the emotion which vibrates at a very low frequency and is regarded as a negative emotion, and the highest being the one which has the highest vibration and is commonly regarded as a positive emotion.

Abraham-Hicks has come up with a series of emotions that will help you work towards feeling better about whatever you are experiencing. Below is their emotional scale, which can be found on page 114 of the book *Ask and It Is Given*.

1. Joy/Appreciation/Empowered/Freedom/Love
2. Passion
3. Enthusiasm/Eagerness/Happiness
4. Positive Expectation/Belief
5. Optimism

6. Hopefulness
7. Contentment
8. Boredom
9. Pessimism
10. Frustration/Irritation/Impatience
11. Overwhelm
12. Disappointment
13. Doubt
14. Worry
15. Blame
16. Discouragement
17. Anger
18. Revenge
19. Hatred/Rage
20. Jealousy
21. Insecurity/Guilt/Unworthiness
22. Fear/Grief/Depression/Despair/Powerlessness

Moving up the scale actually produces a healing effect on the body as each higher vibrating emotion moves you out of stress, struggle, and suffering and into an energy of ease, joy, and abundance.

A lot of personal development / positive thinking schools of thought advise that by going from depression to joy straight away is the way to go. Skip all the other emotions and just fake it till you feel it. What we know today is that this doesn't always work and our bodies actually know when we are not fully feeling the feeling. Sometimes it's just too darn hard to go from rage to love in a heartbeat.

By moving up the scale from, say, fear to rage is actually a healthy thing to do. We cannot suppress our feelings or they become ticking time bombs in our body. They need to be expressed in a healthy way, so by feeling the rage and screaming into your pillow or yelling at the top of your voice in the car on the highway is a great thing to do. It gets it out of you so that you can move on up the scale.

As you continue to feel a more positive feeling, your response to the event or situation changes. No longer does it have the same trigger or pull that it once had. You can think about it now without the sadness or anger overwhelming you. This is the space where miracles can occur. You are now in a position where you can change your perspective. The scale allows room for grace to show up and healing to take place. Forgiveness can be found within the scale and with forgiveness comes transcendence.

If you find yourself stuck in a negative feeling and unable to shift then ask for help, pray, release it to God. It is such a load to bear to journey through life doing everything for yourself. Trust me, I know that well. Releasing emotion to the divine takes the burden off you allowing you the freedom to breathe. Negative emotions are so constricting; all that dark, dense energy trapped inside weighs us down. Life gets hard; our own life force begins to weaken under the pressure.

No-one said you have to carry that alone; who told you it was your burden to bear? Where did you adopt the belief that you couldn't offer up your pain to Source so that divine love could transform you? We don't need to stay stuck in the bottom of the scale. We don't even need to play there; we can live at the top if we continue to evolve and adopt a StressLess life. Where would you rather spend your days? I've spent a lifetime reaching for love, joy, and freedom. I did it the hard way; I struggled for the right for these emotions to be part of me and yet they were mine to own all along.

The more you practise moving to a better healing feeling, the easier it gets. Each time you participate in a selah moment, becoming aware of your emotions, you empower yourself with the gift of choice. You get to choose how you want to feel, you get to choose how you respond to life: that's power, that's freedom, and that's a gift.

CHAPTER 14

Letting Go Of Frustration

One of the biggest blocks to a StressLess life is frustration—constant frustration from wanting something different than what is. I know this so well. Feeling frustrated because my financial situation totally sucked. Annoyed that I wasn't more successful in my business. Irritated that life just kept throwing me curve balls and I kept getting knocked off track.

Frustration is a low vibrating feeling; it attracts lack, pain and struggle. Chronic frustration creates a knot in the body and minimises our life force.

Frustration means the feeling of being annoyed or upset as a result of not being able to change or achieve something. When we think something has to be different than what it currently is, we are in turn saying that something is wrong. When we believe something is wrong we negate any good in the circumstance.

It's like energetically we have created a big hole for ourselves. We have in effect made it harder for ourselves to move forward because we are like a dog paddling around in a pool of negativity and exasperation. The only way to get out of the water is to love what is.

Byron Katie is a master at this. In her body of work called "The Work" she shares how there is a way of questioning and identifying the thoughts which cause anger, fear, and depression, and how to undo these thoughts, allowing the mind to return to its true awakened nature.

I recommend reading her book titled *Loving What Is: How Four Questions can Change your Life* (Random House) as she really gets to the truth of the issue by answering just four questions.

These questions are:

Is this true?

Can you absolutely know that it's true?

How do you react when you think that thought?

Who would you be without the thought?

By working through these questions we realise that basically our thoughts are doing us, not the other way around. When we believe our thoughts instead of what is true for us, we experience stress. She states that we are not disturbed by what happens to us but by our thoughts about what happens to us. The way to end our stress is to investigate the thinking that lies behind it.

When we look into our thoughts we realise that it's not actually the circumstance that is the issue. By accepting what is in the moment we open up a space for grace to step in and take over. Our job is not to push against what is but to soften into it. This is not saying that you don't want it to be different, but there is an allowing for Source to enter. Instead of acting like a dog paddling around frantically trying to stay afloat, we ride the wave and let it choose the path. Sometimes the wave is not the one we would have chosen, but it turns out to be the one where you ended up having the ride of your life.

In addition to our thoughts ruling us, another thing that keeps us from living a StressLess life is not being in truth with our emotions.

I fought against not being able to work and exercise for months. The frustration I felt in my body each time it would give out on me was huge. This is how my self-talk usually went on any given day:

"This is bullshit, I should be able to make it through the day without getting friggin' tired all the time. It's not fair, why is this happening to me? I'm over this crap; I should be able to do what I want to do when I want to do it. This is so frustrating; I have work I want to do and I can't do it because I have no energy. When am I going to get better? It's been months, I should be fine by now!"

Can you feel the energy coming from those thoughts? What I was actually doing was going into my story about disease and illness, and thinking that the feelings I was feeling were bad. This just kept me stuck and on a loop. The emotions kept playing over and over again because I wasn't processing them in a healthy way; I wasn't allowing them to have a voice and be really felt and then released. I was believing my thoughts and not seeing the real issue.

My story grew bigger and bigger in my mind, like a movie; the colours got brighter, the sound got louder, and the emotions got heightened. When we keep reliving something we make it bigger, we exaggerate it until it resembles nothing like the truth.

We need to get out of our head and into our bodies, so that we can remove ourselves from our story, process the emotions in a healthy way, and free ourselves from the stress, struggle, and strain.

When something frustrates you, what is it you say to yourself on a daily basis? What thoughts go through your head? I suggest you write them down. I kept a journal and this was my saving grace. It allowed me to process all my emotions and feel them so that they wouldn't be pushed away or squashed down.

It's not the emotions that are bad; the frustration is not the enemy here. We want to feel the frustration so that it can be released. Carol Tuttle said, "Emotions are like a wave: you need to ride the wave in order to feel them."

By writing in a journal you are riding the wave of emotion without it affecting others. Your frustration or anger is being subjected onto the paper, not your poor, unsuspecting spouse. They are being acknowledged and that is all they want. Emotions are like little parts of us that need to be seen and heard; just like little children, they need our attention.

A great way to do this is to have a dialogue with the part of you that feels the emotion. Below is a transcript of a written dialogue I had with my frustration when I was going through the initial months of adrenal fatigue. I wrote this out using dominant and non-dominant handwriting. This process accesses both sides of the brain: the responses from the non-dominant hand are from the unconscious; they are unfiltered and without ego. The abbreviation for dominant hand is DH and non-dominant hand is NDH.

Integrating disowned parts of yourself

Sitting in a comfortable position, eyes closed for a minute and just going inwards. Breathing deeply and with each breath feeling your body relax deeper and deeper.

Think of the thing that is frustrating you at the moment. Bring it to the front of your mind. The frustration is a part of you—describe this part of you in detail: what age are they; what is their personality; what are they wearing? See in your mind's eye all of the details of this part of you, which is frustrated.

You love this part of you, just like you would your own child; this part of you is just scared, and they want to be seen. They are the disowned parts of you that need to be brought into the light again.

Now have a conversation with them. Ask them why they are frustrated.

DH: How old are you?

NDH: Twenty.

DH: Why are you frustrated?

NDH: I found out a big lie in my family.

DH: How can I support you?

NDH: I don't know.

DH: What are you scared of?

NDH: Not being able to take care of myself.

DH: Why does that scare you?

NDH: I have to take care of myself, I have no one else.

DH: Why do you think that?

NDH: I've been betrayed.

DH: What do you need to do?

NDH: I have to be strong and fend for myself; I can't rely on anyone else.

DH: What do you want from me?

NDH: To be loved just as I am.
DH: I can love you just as you are.
NDH: I want to feel safe.
DH: I will protect you.

I felt my twenty-year-old soften and expand. I felt the fear disappear. The twenty-year-old that had been disowned is now integrated again. She has been so scared for so many years; she just wants to be protected.

It's the parts of us that are not integrated that take over. My whole adult life I felt that I had to work in order to feel safe. I had to be able to look after myself because I felt alone and abandoned. If I couldn't work then I wouldn't be independent, and if I am not independent I would have to rely on others and they would let me down again.

By bringing that twenty-year-old into the light, I could see why I was feeling so frustrated for being sick. It wasn't the fact I was sick as much as the fear that I would lose my independence and have to rely on others, and that was a scary thing because I had been betrayed in the past.

The frustration was masking the fear of the twenty-year-old; it wasn't the forty-five-year-old with adrenal fatigue that was the real issue here. When I saw that I could rely on others I began to let go. I had my husband who was running our other companies; I had my retreat staff working to run the spa. I wasn't that scared, betrayed young woman anymore. Once the fear was addressed I could accept the situation for what it was: a moment to rest my body and restore myself. An opportunity to heal and reveal my higher self.

It was only from embracing this knowing that I felt safe enough to really go deep with my healing. To really be immersed into the moment and suck the marrow out of what life was offering me. A chance to rest and replenish, a chance to be shown love, a chance to know what it feels like to let myself ask for help, and a chance to let my guard down and feel utterly protected and safe.

You can do this process for any emotion or situation that you feel is causing you stress. It may take a few sessions but be patient and persist.

It takes a little while for this part of you to trust again. You wouldn't give up on a child so don't give up on yourself.

If you are not into writing, then dialoguing is just as effective. I have conversations with my emotions all the time. Connecting with a feeling that keeps rearing its head and won't seem to go away is one of the most effective ways I have found to get back onto the Pace of Grace.

Combining this with Byron Katie's four questions always shines the truth on any issue.

These processes are great to do in your selah moments, to be able to give yourself the gift of time. Time to listen to your thoughts and know if they speak the truth. Time to integrate the disowned parts of yourself and move past emotions which are keeping you stuck. Don't let frustration keep you from accessing the Pace of Grace. Don't be a victim to hoodwinked thoughts.

There is inside each and every one of us a part that surrenders to "what is" and knows that everything is as it should be. This part is often shouted down by the unintegrated parts, but it is there, and we can access it using the same method of inner dialogue we spoke of before.

This part is your higher self; it is okay with the sickness within. It is okay with not being able to have a child; it is okay with being single. This part is known as the surrendered part of yourself. The piece of you that knows that it is this or something better. By accessing this part we can claim the peace that is so rightfully ours in any given situation.

To find this inner surrender just practise the written or verbal inner dialogue the same as before. Below is the actual transcript I used for surrendering to my adrenal fatigue.

Transcript for surrendering to adrenal fatigue

Sitting in a comfortable position, eyes closed for a minute and just going inwards. Breathing deeply and with each breath feeling your body relax deeper and deeper.

Begin to become aware of that part of you which is surrendered to having adrenal fatigue, the space where all knowing rests.

DH: Can you feel this place?

NDH: Yes.

DH: What does it feel like?

NDH: Warm, soft and peaceful.

DH: What does it say to you?

NDH: You are going to be okay.

DH: What else?

NDH: Trust in the process; trust that everything is as it should be.

DH: What are you feeling?

NDH: I am scared to.

DH: Why?

NDH: What if I can't trust it?

DH: Is this your twenty-year-old talking?

NDH: Yes.

DH: Tell her you love her and that she is safe.

NDH: I love you, you can trust me and you are safe.

DH: Now can you trust your surrendered part?

NDH: Yes, I trust it.

I had a lot of conversations similar to this because my twenty-year-old kept coming back but the more I persisted the quieter her voice became. The voice of my surrendered place became stronger. It was in the act of complete surrender that I found unconditional love for my situation and myself.

The walls of frustration and fear were knocked down and replaced with a gentleness and a depth of certainty I'd not felt before. Not certainty that the situation will change, but certainty that I will be okay no matter what.

From this place grace is our travelling companion, from this place we can move mountains, and from this place we can change the world.

CHAPTER 15

The Quickest Way To Change Your Beliefs In Order To Release Stress, Struggle and Fatigue

When I was in grade three my parents moved across town, which meant that I had to change schools halfway through the year. For anyone who has had to do this, you can understand that it can be quite traumatic being the new kid on the block.

One week into my traumatic experience, something happened that would change the course of my life for the next twenty years. This one little event, which when I look back now seems so insignificant, managed to instil in me a belief that I was stupid and would never amount to anything.

On this particular day my grade three teacher was providing us with instructions on how to clean out our paper drawers where we held certain assignments we had completed over the term. There were some papers that needed to be placed in the rubbish bin and some we needed to hold on to.

I was obviously not listening and threw out some of the ones I needed to keep. Her reaction to my little cleanout went like this:

She stood me on the stage where she taught from, she put the bin at my feet, and she sat the whole class down in front of me so that I was the centre of attention. She then made me pick out the papers from the bin one by one and proceeded to tell me how dumb I was, and that I must be the stupidest little girl she had ever taught, and how I would never amount to anything if I couldn't learn to listen now.

My whole world as far as I was concerned was laughing at me and I was crying my eyes out. So in my nine-year-old mind, my belief became I must be stupid because she should know, right? She was my teacher, after all.

I went from being a very extroverted, confident little girl to one who would never draw attention to herself. I became very shy and introverted. I stopped trying at school, because what was the point, right? This one event changed my life for the next twenty years.

Conscious self-care is about throwing out those old limiting self-sabotaging beliefs and adopting new beliefs that provide us with a platform to thrive.

Eventually I changed my belief that I was not smart to "I can learn anything if I want to" and from there I started enrolling in every course I could find. I eventually graduated as a nurse, became a personal trainer, started my own business, created an award-winning retreat and day spa, wrote a couple of books and now own a successful international coaching company with my husband. All this from a girl who believed she would never do anything special in her life.

Our beliefs are not set in stone; we can change them in an instant when provided with the right framework and stimulation. I've worked with personal training clients who were overweight and detested exercise, and are now personal trainers themselves. All they did was just change one little belief which then created a ripple effect.

If you look behind what is stressing you out right now and what is your biggest struggle you will find certain beliefs associated with this stress. For example, I was so scared of public speaking that if I had to get up in front of a crowd it would stress me out days before the event. It was becoming so bad that it was stopping me from really getting out there and making a difference in my business at the time as a personal trainer. I knew if I could speak to an audience, I would be able to influence a lot more people but I was just so darned scared to step out of my comfort zone.

When I took the time to look at what the belief was behind this fear what came up was: "If I stand up in front of a crowd I will be humiliated". When I went deeper into this belief I saw that nine-year-old girl being laughed at on a stage whilst her teacher humiliated her.

As an adult I realised that this belief was no longer serving me and preventing me from reaching my highest potential. As I shone awareness on it, the light was able to transcend that fear and I could move into a space of doing it scared. In this place I could allow myself to feel the fear and do it anyway.

I did this for years, with lots of limiting beliefs, and I was getting by; then one day I came across a technique which could literally remove the fear and stress from my body within a few minutes. Instead of taking years, I could now move through stuck energy so quickly it was life transforming.

This technique is called Emotional Freedom technique or EFT. If you have been into personal development for a while you may have already heard about it and have been using it successfully. If you are new to it then I urge you to check out www.thetappingsolution.com Nick and Jessica Ortner have done amazing work in this area, and have a wealth of information there for you to learn and start implementing right now. Below is an overview of Emotional Freedom Technique adapted from the tapping solution website.

Basically EFT is a type of meridian tapping that combines ancient Chinese acupressure and modern psychology with amazing results. Tapping utilises the body's energy meridian points by stimulating them with your fingertips—literally tapping into your body's own energy and healing power. From pain relief to weight loss, tapping is proving to be a powerful, well-researched, and easy-to-learn-and-apply technique.

When you're experiencing a negative emotional state such as anger or fear, your brain goes on alert. It prepares your body to enter a full-blown, fight-or-flight response. All the body's defence systems are turned on to support either fighting or fleeing from the danger. Your adrenaline pumps, your muscles tense, and your blood pressure, heart rate, and blood sugar all rise to give you extra energy to meet the challenge. Most of our fight-or-flight responses today are triggered internally rather than from a physical challenge such as running from a crazy psychopath. For many of us, the internally generated stress response is triggered by a negative memory or thought that has its roots in past trauma or conditioned learning from childhood. What tapping does is halt the fight-or-flight response and reprogram the brain and body to act and react differently.

The stress response begins in your brain in the almond-shaped amygdala, one of the components of the limbic system, or midbrain. The midbrain is located between the frontal lobes (the cortex) and the hindbrain (also called the reptilian brain—the earliest, most primitive part of the brain). The limbic system is the source of emotions and long-term memory, and it's where negative experiences are encoded. It signals the brain to mobilise the body in the fight-or-flight response. Tapping on the meridian endpoints helps to deactivate the amygdala's alarm and sends a calming response to the body, and the amygdala recognises that it's safe.

The basic technique requires you to focus on the negative emotion at hand: a fear or anxiety, a bad memory, or any other aspect around an unresolved problem, or anything that's bothering you. While maintaining your mental focus on this issue, use your fingertips to tap five to seven times each on nine of the body's meridian points mentioned below. Tapping on these meridian points—while concentrating on accepting and resolving the negative emotion—will access your body's energy, restoring it to a balanced state.

Meridians are simply energy, which circulates through your body along a specific network of channels. You can tap into this energy at any point along the system. This concept comes from the doctrines of traditional Chinese medicine, which referred to the body's energy as 'chi'. In ancient times, the Chinese discovered one hundred meridian points. They also discovered that by stimulating these meridian points, they could heal.

In some ways, tapping is similar to acupuncture. Like tapping, acupuncture achieves healing through stimulating the body's meridians and energy flow. However, unlike acupuncture, tapping involves no needles. Tapping is simple and painless. It can be learned by anyone. And you can apply it to yourself, whenever you want, wherever you are. It's less expensive and less time consuming. It can be used with specific emotional intent towards your own unique life challenges and experiences.

An exciting set of research studies was undertaken by Dr Dawson Church. His team performed a randomised controlled trial to study how an hour-long tapping session would impact the stress levels of eighty-three subjects. To do this, Dr Church and his team measured their level of cortisol, a hormone secreted by the body when it undergoes stress. Their findings were that the average level of cortisol reduction was 24 percent, with a whopping reduction of almost 50 percent in some subjects! In comparison, there was no significant cortisol reduction in those who underwent an hour of traditional talk therapy. Dr Church also created The Stress Project, which teaches tapping to war veterans suffering with PTSD. The results have been astounding: an average 63 percent decrease in PTSD symptoms after six rounds of tapping.

As discussed, tapping can be used for everything—try it on everything! In this example, we'll focus on general stress.

Try it now with this initial sequence. Here's how a basic tapping sequence works:

- Identify the problem you want to focus on. It can be general stress, or it can be a specific situation or issue, which causes you to feel stressed.
- Consider the problem or situation. How do you feel about it right now? Rate the intensity level of your anxiety, with zero being the lowest level of anxiety and ten being the highest.
- Compose your set-up statement. Your set-up statement should acknowledge the problem you want to deal with, and then follow it with an unconditional affirmation of yourself as a person.

"Even though I feel this stress, I deeply and completely accept myself."

"Even though I'm nervous about speaking in public, I deeply and completely accept myself."

"Even though I'm feeling this anxiety about my relationship, I deeply and completely accept myself."

"Even though I panic when I think about _____, I deeply and completely accept myself."

"Even though I'm worried about how to pay the bills this month, I deeply and completely accept myself."

Perform the set-up

With four fingers on one hand, tap the Karate Chop point on your other hand. The Karate Chop point is on the outer edge of the hand, on the opposite side from the thumb.

Repeat the set-up statement three times aloud, while simultaneously tapping the Karate Chop point. Now take a deep breath!

Get ready to begin tapping! Here are some tips to help you achieve the right technique.

You should use a firm but gentle pressure.

You can use all four fingers, or just the first two (the index and middle fingers). Four fingers are generally used on the top of the head, the collarbone, under the arm, or wider areas. On sensitive areas, like around the eyes, you can use just two.

Tap with your fingertips, not your fingernails.

The tapping order begins at the top and works down. You can end by returning to the top of the head, to complete the loop.

Now, tap five to seven times each on the remaining eight points in the following sequence:

Eyebrow

The inner edges of the eyebrows, closest to the bridge of the nose. Use two fingers.

Side of eye

The hard area between the eye and the temple. Use two fingers. Feel out this area gently so you don't poke yourself in the eye!

Under eye

The hard area under the eye, that merges with the cheekbone. Use two fingers, in line beneath the pupil.

Under nose

The point centred between the bottom of the nose and the upper lip. Use two fingers.

Chin

This point is right beneath the previous one, and is centred between the bottom of the lower lip and the chin.

Collarbone

Tap just below the hard ridge of your collarbone with four fingers.

Underarm

On your side, about four inches beneath the armpit. Use four fingers.

Head

The crown, centre, and top of the head. Tap with all four fingers on both hands.

And back where you started, to complete the sequence. As you tap on each point, repeat a simple reminder phrase, such as "my stress" or "my finances".

Now take another deep breath!

Now that you've completed the sequence, focus on your problem again. How intense is the anxiety now, in comparison to a few minutes ago? Give it a rating on the same number scale. If your anxiety is still higher than two, you can do another round of tapping. Keep tapping until the anxiety is gone. Now that you've focused on dispelling your immediate anxiety, you can work on installing some positive feelings instead.

This approach is different from traditional "positive thinking". You're not being dishonest with yourself. You're not trying to obscure the stress and anxiety inside yourself with insincere affirmations. Rather, you've confronted and dealt with the anxiety and negative feelings, offering deep and complete acceptance to both your feelings and yourself. Now, you're turning your thoughts and vibrations to the powerful and positive. It's not just a mental trick; instead, you're using these positive phrases and tapping to tune into the very real energy of positivity, affirmation, and joy that is implicit inside you. You're actually changing your body's energy into a more positive flow, a more positive vibration.

Here are some example phrases to guide you:

I am becoming a more calm and peaceful person.

I love who I am becoming.

I enjoy the feeling of peace inside me.

I am becoming joyful and full of hope.

I have faith that everything will turn out right.

EFT moves stuck energy through and out of our system so that we can move forward. I encourage you to do a couple of minutes each day when first starting out and increase this if you feel something coming up which needs to be addressed. It is a great tool to incorporate into your selah time as well. Have fun with it; these tools may seem simple but the profound is found in simplicity. We make things far too complicated and this only adds to our stressful, busy lives.

CHAPTER 16

Stress Bomb, Stress Bomb, You're My Stress Bomb

One of the things that surprised me most when I was told that I had adrenal fatigue was that it was a stress-related issue. I had prided myself on thinking I was not a stressful person. I believed that I didn't have a lot of stress in my life. I wasn't an anxious or overly jumpy type. I wasn't prone to moments of intense anger. I reacted calmly under pressure.

What I came to realise is that a person can appear to be cool, calm, and collected on the surface yet internally their organs and systems of the body can be completely overworked and run down.

Because of my driven personality type and the way I always pushed at life I had spun my little adrenals up into a tizzy and they had run out of Jing.

We talked about how the Jing energy rests and sits in our kidney and adrenal meridian. Jing is about that primordial life force energy. It's the energy that keeps you going long after you thought you should stop. It is that deep will to survive and it is all about nourishing that primordial life force essence, and I was depleted.

In my mind I imagined a thousand little dark balls all clinging on to my kidneys and adrenals, and they were blocking the flow of energy and sapping me of mine. I have come to term these little balls stress bombs.

I like to imagine the blocks to ease, joy, and abundance as little stress bombs. Each time we eat something that causes inflammation in our body, every time we think a negative thought, suppress an emotion, get anxious, or overwhelmed we create little stress bombs which get fired into our bodies and land somewhere in our energy system or our physical systems.

They then get stuck there until we do something to move them like change our diet, deal with an issue that is bothering us, experience forgiveness, or go back and heal old wounds.

When we continue to think the same thought, eat the same foods, experience the same negative emotions, the little stress bombs land on that same area and start to stack up causing the vibration in this area to alter. The response to the stress bomb build-up can range from blocks to manifesting money, attracting bad relationships, or experiencing lots of hardship in certain areas of your life. It is also when we start to experience signs of disease and illness. This is where cancer begins, or heart disease or diabetes.

The cells in this area are reacting to the different vibration and either atrophying or morphing into something else.

It's like if we couldn't get blood flow to our feet we would be in major risk of amputation. Without blood flow our feet would be cut off from their life force. It is the same with the energy systems in our body. If we have stress bombs along the pathways or in our chakras then we are blocking the energy flow for that related pathway.

In chapter 9 I explain how to add the nourishment back to our adrenals and rebuild our Jing energy. Another way I helped my body clear the stress bombs is with guided meditations.

I love the work of Doreen Virtue and her book *Archangels & Ascended Masters*, Hay House, 2007 describes the attributes of each angel and master and how we can ask for help for anything we need.

Guided visualisation for removing stress bombs

Sit back and get comfortable. Take a deep breath in and as you slowly breathe out feel any tension in your body release and soften. Breathe in deeply again and now scan your body from head to toe, noticing any signs of tightness and tension. Breathing slowly and deeply and with each exhale feel your body relax completely.

As we begin this meditation know that you are completely safe and at any time if you feel uncomfortable you can simply open your eyes and come back into the room safely.

Now we evoke Archangel Raphael and Archangel Michael to join us for this clearing. Please surround us with your loving powerful presence.

Imagine yourself walking in a beautiful green meadow. The sun is shining down on you, warming your body from the inside out. There is a gentle breeze blowing. The sky is a brilliant blue, and you can see miles and miles of gently swaying trees and grass.

You come across a golden gate, and you open it and step through. You see a big beautiful tree and decide to lie down underneath it. A bed of soft grass cushions your body, and as you begin to close your eyes and relax you feel the powerful healing presence of Archangels Michael and Raphael around you.

You feel safe and loved, and as you lie here begin to scan your body from the top of your head to your toes. Notice for any signs of stress bombs. You may see them with your mind's eye, sense them or even feel them in your body. They appear darker and the energy is dense; they may also differ in size and shape.

If you see them do not be alarmed, simply send them light and love. There is nothing to fear. Look or feel around your head, coming down into your throat, spreading out over your shoulders. Down your arms into your hands and fingers. See your chest and stomach, your hips and pelvis area. Coming down into your thighs, your shins and into your ankles, feet and toes.

Bringing your attention back up into your calves, your hamstrings, your buttocks, into your lower back, middle and upper back, noticing your spine. Then sensing for any small dark shapes in your neck, the back of your head.

You may notice many darker shapes of varying sizes. There may be clusters in a certain area. Remember, do not be afraid: these stress bombs are simply signals for us to pay attention.

Now imagine an elixir of white light coming into your body via your head. This elixir feels warm and comforting. See the light travelling through your body dissolving all stress bombs in its path.

See it travel down from your head, neck, shoulders, lighting up everything in its path.

This light is your healing light; it has the power to completely remove all stress bombs. As you watch it filling your body you see the black spots disappearing before your very eyes. You feel cleansed and purified.

You feel your cells and organs come alive, expand, and cleanse.

Continue this until your whole body has been filled with this beautiful elixir of healing white light.

You begin to feel light; you are bathing in this beautiful white crystal light that is being pumped into your whole body.

Please thank Archangels Raphael and Michael for this healing, cleansing process. As you continue to breathe you become aware of your surroundings once again. You see the magnificent tree sheltering you and feel the grass cushioning your body.

You allow a big stretch, and slowly get up and walk back to the golden gate; you step through and now you are back in your room, sitting in your chair or lying down in this present moment. Allow a nice deep breath and then gently open your eyes.

This guided meditation can be used whenever you feel like you are blocked or need to cleanse or detox. I find it a wonderful addition to the other tools and processes I share with you in this book for clearing away blocks caused by stress.

Please note though that if you do not make any changes the stress bombs will return. This is not a quick fix. Stress needs to be addressed emotionally, mentally, physically, and energetically in order for you to live a StressLess life.

Over time, with commitment and desire, you will see your life changing. You will feel the difference in your body. You will hear the words coming from your mouth changing. Life will feel lighter, more energetic. What once was the cause of your heartache is a distant memory. Your desire for junk food is replaced with a need for living, soul-enriching foods. Your taste buds have literally changed.

This way of living is your birthright. It is available for each and every one of us if we choose it. My desire is you lose the stress bombs from your life and begin to smother yourself with love bombs. Big, beautiful, crazy, wild love bombs. I'm sending you one from my heart to yours right now; can you feel it?

CHAPTER 17

Stopping Phantom Stress

In my early thirties I accepted an invitation from a friend to housesit his country cottage in a tiny town about thirty minutes from where I was living at the time.

The cottage was the cutest thing I had ever seen with a grapevine-covered veranda which swept around the whole house. There was a cosy fireplace and the nearest neighbour was a five-minute drive.

On my very first night I remember being so excited by the thought of having a space for just myself and my little dog to relax and have some uninterrupted solitude.

After spending a beautiful day resting by the fire, reading a great book, going for walks around the paddocks and cooking up a wonderful meal, I retired to bed early.

No sooner had I turned off the light than I heard footsteps walking on the wooden floorboards of the porch. My heart was in my mouth and my whole body just tightened. My nervous system was on full alert. Danger, Will Robinson, danger. As I held my breath, the footsteps got closer and closer to the end of the house where my bedroom was. I suddenly remembered the butcher's knife in the kitchen by the oven. With as much courage as I could muster I slunk out of bed and slid across the floor, combat style, grabbed the knife, and caterpillared back to my bed. It is amazing how all the moves you have ever watched in the movies come back to keep you safe.

As the footsteps got louder and louder, and my need to lose control of all bodily functions got stronger and stronger, I prayed to every higher power I could think of, from God to the fairies in the garden; I wasn't being picky.

Then as the steps reached my window, a huge knock on the glass did me in. My whole life flashed before my eyes; this was how I was going to die, really? Single, housesitting in the middle of nowhere, with my dog in my bed?

After what seemed like five minutes of not breathing I had not heard any other noises. Had he gone or was he at my front door, jimmying the lock? I don't know if it was an overdose of cortisol or lack of oxygen to the brain but after an hour of silence, I managed to fall asleep.

In the morning I opened my eyes, and said an instant prayer of gratitude that I had survived and was here to live another day. I went outside to search for any signs left behind by my would-be killer. What I found was a trail of animal droppings leading to my bedroom window. After glancing in the corner of the windowsill I noticed a huge Bogong moth.

My spider senses were tingling; I stepped off the porch and as I turned the corner I came face to face with a huge kangaroo, staring me down. Then it hit me like a lightning bolt. My would-be killers were a kangaroo and a Bogong moth.

I share this story because in reality what stresses us out is often our own imagination; rarely is it the truth. I call it phantom stress. The only thing is our bodies can't tell the difference. When we journey into the future we cannot predict the outcome, all we are doing is imagining different scenarios. If it makes you happy then keep imagining it; if it stresses you out then STOP IT.

Gavin's story

In my work as a wellness coach I hear stories all the time of how people have ventured into the future, imagined a frightening scenario, and this is keeping them stuck, unable to heal, and diminishing their full power.

One gentleman that comes to mind is Gavin. Gavin has Crohn's disease and is unable to work. Years of operations and treatments to help him be able to live with the disease functionally and return to work have not helped, and Gavin is now depressed and shut down.

When I asked Gavin what happens when he experiences pain he said that in his mind he imagines that he will have to go back to hospital and have another operation. This frightens him and makes the pain even more excruciating.

The fact that he goes to the worst-possible scenario does Gavin no favours. It is the thing that is preventing his recovery because he is re-living an experience from his past which was traumatic for him.

We gave Gavin a combination of natural pain relief techniques, which he could use whenever he was experiencing pain. Then we also worked on suggesting that Gavin get out of his head and focus on breathing through the pain. Acknowledging that the pain is there and going deeper into it. Asking questions to the pain such as, "What is it you are trying to tell me?" and "What is it you want me to do?"

What Gavin is doing when he focuses on the pain and asking the questions is acknowledging that it is there, not trying to suppress it and push it down, and seeing what emotion is behind the pain. When we understand the emotion we can begin the healing work of clearing the pain.

Asking the question in combination with the natural pain relief techniques such as breath work and Emotional Freedom Technique keeps him out of the future and in the present. His mind cannot take over and it is in the present moment where all power is.

It is common for our thoughts to go into the future and imagine new possibilities. This is how dreams are created and desires formed. The imagination is a powerful tool for manifestation, but I say if we don't like what we are imagining then don't go there.

Abraham Hicks says that if we focus on something for seventeen seconds we start to become a matching vibration to it. Do it for sixty-eight seconds and it can become our reality *(Ask and It Is Given, page 109)*. That's awesome if we are focusing on things that make us happy, but how often do we put our attention on the negative? How often are we focusing on our disease, our diagnosis, our relationship horribilis, or our negative bank balance?

No wonder we keep living the same day over and over; it's because we keep thinking the same thoughts over and over, and most of these thoughts come from our imagined future, which is not real

.

Vibrational breathing

A process I use for coming back from a wicked vision in my imagination and remembering what is real is what I call vibrational breathing. It is a deep breath followed by a loud exhale which sounds like a sigh.

Basically how it works is that the exhale stimulates the vagus nerve, which is at the centre of our emotional brain or lymbric brain, to release oxytocin into our body. This then puts us back into the parasympathetic nervous system and into rest and digest, and out of the sympathetic nervous system, which is our fight, flight or freeze response.

When our thoughts go into worst-possible scenario, we start to feel the negative emotions associated with this image and our bodies don't know that it is not real. It thinks, "Holy smoke, Batman, this is bad; we need to run," and produces adrenalin and noradrenalin and cortisol which courses through our bloodstream, enabling us to flee from the imagined image we have just played out in our minds.

That is the reason why so many of us are tired and wired now; our bodies are on continual high alert because we operate from the worst-possible scenario so often and consume thoughts which are not true.

When I notice any feelings of stress in my body, such as tightness, contraction, or tension, I allow a vibrational breath, enabling my nervous system to align itself back into its restful state. This reminds me to change my thoughts and come back to the present moment.

Vibrational breathing technique

Have your mouth slightly open with a little smile dancing on your lips.

Shoulders are relaxed and your rib cage is open.

Allow a deep breath with a pleasurable exhale.

Do this every time you feel stressed; I guarantee it will work wonders.

Lose the guilt and the "what ifs"

Another thing that makes us stressed is guilt from living in the past. The only thing living with guilt ever achieves is a sore neck from looking back all the time. I have firsthand experience with this as I lived with guilt for a very long time before I learnt this lesson.

I owned a golf buggy; we used it at our spa and retreat and every day when I collected the mail I would take the buggy as the driveway was long and steep. My dogs, Diggity and Delhi, loved to race the buggy up the hill. Diggity could usually beat it but Delhi is half his size so she would always be running behind, tongue hanging out with a big smile on her face.

One day I saw that Diggity was right beside me and as I looked behind me for Delhi I suddenly felt a huge bump; Diggity was nowhere to be seen. My heart was in my throat as I realised he was under the buggy.

As I got out I saw his little white paw sticking out from under the wheel; as I bent down to look under I noticed that his whole body was under the front tyre. He was alive, just looking up at me, his little brown eyes saying, "WTF, Mum!"

I tried to lift the buggy off him but it was far too heavy. Diggity weighs ten kilograms, it weighs nearly five hundred kilograms; even my husband can't lift it. The next few moments I cannot remember, but looking back I now believe that my angels were with me in full force because all of a sudden the buggy lifted, Diggity was freed, and I was racing him up to my car to take him to the veterinary hospital.

The vet searched him all over and could not find any broken bones but I was to watch him overnight and make sure that he had no internal damage.

The next morning as the vet was checking him, he was amazed that there were not even any bruises on his body. There was not one mark or scratch on him; I, however, had massive bruises on my thighs where I had taken the weight of the golf car.

What I found myself doing weeks and months after the incident was re-enacting the whole event with different what-ifs added in to increase the drama intensity. What if it was Delhi, she is so much smaller? What if he had died? What if it had been worse? What if I couldn't get the buggy off him? All these imagined "what ifs" were causing me major stress. Yet I felt I couldn't stop, my mind just went there at random times during the day and in my dreams.

What I eventually realised was that I was holding on to the guilt because I hadn't forgiven myself. It was an accident, and I was beating myself up. I wasn't focused on the miracle of what happened; I was paying attention to the imagined untruths which were keeping me from being able to fully show up in this moment.

Forgiveness crystallises the calcification caused by guilt and living in the "what ifs". I had to forgive myself completely, and I needed to ask God for help because this was too big for me to do alone. My dogs are my babies; to me they are just as valuable as the people in my life.

Every time I thought about it, I released it to God and said the words, "I forgive you, Karina, I love you." The more I did this, the less frequent the memory came up. Now, the only time I think about it is if I share the story with someone in order for me to provide an example of how guilt is a shitty thing to hang on to.

If guilt is something that causes you stress and pain then I encourage you to release it to a higher power, whether you call it God, or Buddha or the angels, whatever it is for you. Ask for help and then practise forgiving yourself.

If you are continually asking "What if?" to something that happened in the past then I beg you, STOP. It is not serving you in any way, shape, or form.

If your thoughts are keeping you in a low vibrational state then stop TRYING to change them and just do it. Remember, just think a higher vibrating thought for seventeen seconds. Then think another and ponder on this for seventeen seconds. Keep doing this for as little as sixty-eight seconds and you will begin to actualise these thoughts into reality.

Then ask yourself, what is the kangaroo and Bogong moth in my life? What do I fear that is coming from my imagination? Where is the phantom stress that makes me feel anxious, fearful, or powerless? What is keeping me from truly living a StressLess life?

I think this calls for a selah moment, don't you?

CHAPTER 18

Sign Of The Pace Of Grace

Whenever I feel that I am in the energy of stress, struggle, and fatigue and knocked off the path to the Pace of Grace, which happens most days, I perform what I call the sign of the Pace of Grace. In the beginning I started placing my hands in the area of each of these points on my body to remind myself where I am out of alignment.

This ritual reminded me of the Catholic blessing for the sign of the cross so I called mine the Pace of Grace sign. It involves simply touching or placing your hand over the forehead, heart, stomach, and pelvic bone regions.

The points are the forehead between the eyes, the heart, the stomach, and the base of the spine or root chakra. By performing this sign, it reminds us to ask a series of questions related to each position. We are then able to determine the correct course of action we need to take in order to get out of stress, struggle, and fatigue, and back into alignment.

The importance of staying in alignment is significant because it is here where external circumstances don't take you out of the game. You are strong, grounded, able to make wiser choices, and are non-reactive and responsive to your surroundings and internal guidance system.

When we place our hand on our forehead in between our eyes, this is our third eye, the place of spiritual insight. When focusing here we ask the following questions:

    1. Have I meditated today?

2. Have I prayed today and asked God for help?
3. Can I see a higher reason or am I open to a higher reason why this is happening?
4. What is the lesson I need to learn?

By answering these questions we are enlisting the help of the divine. Sometimes life is too hard to handle everything on our own; by asking for help from a higher source it becomes more about if it is to be it is up to WE, rather than it is up to ME. That's a huge weight off anyone's shoulders.

Next we touch our heart area and ask the following questions:

1. Am I thinking loving thoughts or fearful thoughts?
2. Am I judging this situation or person?
3. Am I trying to control this situation?
4. Am I accepting that everything is as it should be in this moment?
5. Do I need to choose forgiveness?

By asking ourselves these five questions we can determine if we are coming from a place of love, not fear. When you boil it down to the nitty-gritty, all stress comes from fear. The *Course in Miracles* says that there are only two emotions: love or fear. Anything that is not love is not real. By judging someone you are making them wrong, telling yourself that there has been a wrongdoing, causing emotions such as anger, righteousness, and blame. Negative emotions such as these cause our vibration to slow down, we start to create stress bombs in our body, we operate in struggle and strain, and lack mode. If we don't do something to rectify this it becomes a vicious downward spiral.

When placing our hand on our stomach we ask ourselves the following four questions:

1. What did I eat for breakfast?
2. Have I been consuming a lot of foods which cause inflammation?
3. Have I been nourishing my body?
4. Have I been consuming a StressLess diet?

These four questions will tell you a lot about your state of being in that particular moment. If you have had a coffee and a donut for breakfast then you have peaked your sugar and caffeine intake. Your body is sending out all kinds of hormones to deal with the shock and you wonder why you just lost it with the retail assistant who accidentally overcharged you at the checkout. By starting your day with nourishing, soul-enriching food you are far more likely to respond with kindness when something annoying happens because your cells are basking in the love; your body is aligned with its natural state and sending out lots of feel-good hormones.

Lastly we place our hand in front of the bottom of the pelvis or the root chakra area. The questions we ask are:

1. Have I performed a chakra balancing meditation lately?
2. Did I do my energy medicine techniques this morning?
3. When was the last time I participated in selah time?
4. Have I been dealing with any negative emotions on a regular basis or just letting it build up?
5. Do I need to do a stress bomb cleanse?

These questions relate to our energetic field, and if we suddenly find ourselves overwhelmed or fatigued then the answers may point you in the area you need to go in order to get back to full energy and passion.

Sign of the Pace of Grace in action

Here is how the sign of the Pace of Grace works in action. I mentioned in chapter 1 how before I was diagnosed with adrenal fatigue my husband had informed me that we were likely to lose one of our companies and could be liable for hundreds of thousands of dollars. When he first told me that I remember I didn't freak out; I just needed to know the facts first. How had this happened, what is the worst-case scenario, what is the best? I learnt that our accountant had provided us with incorrect information in relation to our tax situation and because we had not acted by the due date our company was being forced into receivership. My husband had hoped to rectify this situation before I knew anything about it because he didn't want me to worry. Unfortunately the taxman was not playing nice anymore and he could no longer avoid letting me know what was about to go down.

Over the following weeks I started to get really stressed; the more I thought about it and imagined what could potentially happen, what we could lose, it just started to freak me out further. I found myself spiralling into this pit of blame, shame, and despair. I couldn't sleep; I couldn't eat. I was distancing myself from Ian because I blamed him for not telling me and getting us into this mess. I was supposed to be resting and reducing my stress in order to repair my body, and all I was doing was getting sicker and sicker.

I needed to get myself out of this funk I was in fast so I went into selah hibernation and the result was the creation of the questions for the sign of the Pace of Grace. It was in asking myself these questions that I was able to come back from financial ruin so much stronger, wiser, and compassionate than ever before.

Let's review how the questions for each part of the Pace of Grace sign applied to my stressful situation.

In relation to the forehead:

1. Have I meditated today?
2. Have I prayed today and asked God for help?
3. Is there a higher reason this is happening?
4. What is the lesson I need to learn?

It was through continual meditation that I was able to completely heal and restore my body. I am 100 percent certain that if I had not taken up this practice I would still be having a nap every afternoon, and this book would not be in existence. Through meditation I was able to calm my nervous system and let go of the thoughts in my mind. Just twenty minutes a day was enough for me to find reprieve from the fear that was gripping me.

There was no way that I could have handled that situation without the wisdom and insight that I received along the way. In my own human strength I was burnt out; I couldn't even find the energy to have a dream in my heart anymore. There was no energy left over in my own strength to survive a marriage crisis but with the help of God I was carried through on the wings of angels. He was my strength and my support.

For me, I have to believe that there is a higher reason for everything because if I don't then I just get depressed wondering why people have to go through such sadness and grief. Hindsight is an amazing thing because when I look back over my life I can totally see the blessing in the sewer pit. Have you ever looked back over your life and woven a golden thread around all of the pieces that so beautifully appear once you see the link? Oh, if I had have gone here I wouldn't have met that person, and if I had have gotten this dream I wouldn't have this dream, and so on. Each one of our lives is a tapestry of miracles, made up of tears, laughter, and divine right timing.

Lessons are there to be learned in any situation. They make all our failures and mistakes forgivable because once we learn the lesson we don't have to repeat it again. There were so many lessons which came out of losing our company. In taking responsibility for any part I played I was able to take back my power. I was no longer a victim; I could grow and evolve from this and come back stronger. There is always some situation which wants to teach us, mould us, and shape us into the image of our greatest potential.

The questions for my heart point were:
1. Am I thinking loving thoughts or fearful thoughts?
2. Am I judging this situation or person?
3. Am I trying to control this situation?
4. Am I accepting that everything is as it should be in this moment?
5. Do I need to choose forgiveness?

I was so full of fear and uncertainty that it totally ruled the thoughts I was thinking and my actions. It is scary when you don't know if you are going to have a roof over your head in a few weeks' time. But once again all my thoughts were in the future; I was imagining the worst possible outcomes. I had to get out of the future and put all my attention into my heart space. As I would breathe from this place I would just concentrate on love. In that moment, everything was okay, I was safe; from that place I could be happy, I could find peace. My thoughts turned to joy, love, and gratefulness.

In judging Ian and the accountant, I was deflecting any responsibility for my part. Judgement made them wrong but that didn't make me feel any better. There is cause and effect; there are always repercussions and knowing this helped me shift from this all-consuming tightness in my body to a release. I didn't need to make Ian feel any guiltier than what he was already feeling. The energy of judging another and making them wrong has a dark, negative pull downwards attached to it. What happened happened; I couldn't change it. It serves no one to play the blame-and-shame game. If I was to keep going down that road, I could guarantee you I wouldn't be married today.

I remember we started to control how things would play out; if we could just manipulate this then this would happen, or if we just did this then that would happen. That is all fine and good but when it didn't go our way, we became desolate. Instant deflation: it would completely affect our mood and state of being. There are things in life we just can't control; we can do everything in our power to help achieve our desired outcome but when things are not in our power we need to release the attachment to the outcome. Surrender and trust that whatever happens you will be okay. When the group appointed by the liquidator came and took the office furniture owned by that company there was nothing I could do. We couldn't pay back the money we owed so they had to sell off the assets. It was accepting that everything is as it should be that was the thing that got me through. I lived in the know that what does not kill us makes us stronger. We will rebuild from this. For the moment we are not destitute, living on the streets; there are people far worse off than us. This was isolated to just one of our companies; the sky was not actually falling. This quiet strength can get us through anything; it has been the common theme for every story where people have risen up from the ashes and survived the storms of life.

Forgiveness is the salve that heals all wounds. Without it, our souls will fester and bleed out. I made a choice every day to forgive because I knew that if I didn't I would never make it out the other side perfect, whole, and complete.

The stomach point questions were the ones that assisted in keeping up my physical strength and making it through the day without collapsing.

1.   What did I eat for breakfast?
2.   Have I been consuming a lot of foods which cause inflammations?
3.   Have I been nourishing my body?
4.   Have I been consuming a StressLess diet?

My superhero green smoothie became my lifesaver here because stress for me diminishes my appetite, so by having a smoothie in the morning I knew I was probably getting more nourishment for breakfast than most people get in an entire day.

When we eat foods which cause inflammation our bodies need to go into overdrive just to digest this. When your body is compromised to begin with, there is not much energy or life force left over to deal with your emotional crisis. The cleaner I got physically, the greater capacity I had for handling the stress associated with losing the company.

Nourishing my body with clean, green, and conscious foods gave me the strength I needed to stay calm, and not react to situations and events. This way of eating soon became my StressLess diet, which I include in chapter 8. I was able to build up my immune system so that I wasn't susceptible to bugs and parasites because my body was so compromised and in a state of stress.

And lastly the root chakra point questions:

1.   Have I performed a chakra balancing meditation lately?
2.   Did I do my energy medicine techniques this morning?
3.   When was the last time I participated in selah time?
4.   Have I been dealing with any negative emotions on a regular basis or just letting it build up?

There was a lot going on emotionally for me at that time and our chakras are affected by our emotions. When our chakras become blocked or compromised it cuts off our life force from running through our bodies. I had very little life force running through me as it was, so I needed to do all I could to keep what was there flowing. Performing a chakra-clearing meditation helped me to do this, as well as release any stored-up unprocessed emotions.

The energy clearing and protecting techniques which I share in this book assisted in helping me to stay strong, especially when fear and doubt were on the playing field. I found I was able to shield myself from a lot of the negative energy that was happening around me at the time.

My selah times were my saving grace. They provided deep understanding and compassion to the situation. I was able to process my emotions without being judged, and I was able to gain such an enormous amount of insight and perspective. I could not have gotten through it without giving myself the gift of a selah moment.

I have designed a beautiful little card with the questions written on it so that you can print it out and keep it in your bag or at your desk— somewhere handy so that at any time when you know you're stressing out you can just whip it out and take five minutes to do the sign of the Pace of Grace, and get yourself back into alignment a whole lot quicker.

Just go to www.karinastephens.com/pog-gifts

CHAPTER 19

Revolution Through Evolution

"We have to become the best version of ourselves we can be, that is our sacred human contract"
Albert Einstein.

How right you were, Mr Einstein; to live the most ethical lives we can is the key to a kinder world. Lyn White from Animals Australia said, "If we make decisions based on compassion, mercy and selflessness it will lead to choices that do not cause harm to others, human or otherwise."

When we devote our lives to becoming the best version of ourselves, we undertake the most extraordinary adventure imaginable.

Awareness is power: it provides us with the power to change, yet if we are not aware of why we do what we do even though we know what we know, how can we even think to make an impact on this world in our lifetime?

Emotions and feelings are there to guide us home, to our inner home. Yet we tend to ignore or suppress the ones that make us feel less than great. We don't like to go there because we fear what the answer may be. Purpose-based leaders are the ones that go there because they know that when you shine a light on the darkness it disappears.

When we do the inner work then the outer work is magnified. When we break through limiting beliefs and sabotaging habits we have the key to unlock our genius. What used to stress us out no longer bothers us. We play a bigger game and in doing so we have the potential to create a larger impact on the world.

The documentary Unity by director Shaun Monson explores humanity's hopeful transformation from living by killing into living by loving. It is a unique film about compassion for all beings, or all expressions of life going beyond all separation based on form and beyond perceiving opposites.

The world is calling us to wake up and step into our light. To express the truth of who we are in the service of what we are called to do. What if we didn't let fear, stress, and fatigue slow us down? Where would you be if you had more than enough energy to make it through your day? And what if that day involved you doing something that helped heal our planet in some small but significant way?

Imagine putting voice and action to your calling because you overcame the struggle involved in reaching that calling. Think of how amazing it will feel when you achieve your desires because you decided to become the best version of yourself possible.

We create a revolution by change, by saying enough is enough. Revolution needs to come from evolution. Meaning we need to evolve and grow and raise our vibration, and as we do we become the empowered beings capable of creating change in this world.

If anything, I think that what we have learnt by today's fast-food, fast-paced, ASAP rat race is that it's not really working for us. We are more stressed out than ever before. Our planet has never been in such a state of dis-ease, our animals are suffering and I believe it has never been more important to wake up and do something.

According to Dr Lissa Rankin, the average person experiences over **fifty stress events per day** and each one taxes your adrenals and kidneys, leading to eventual fatigue or worse, *disease*. In order to create change, we have to be the change we want to create. We must become the type of person we need to be in order to inspire others to do the same. Then together we can revolutionise the things we care about.

As we take the time to work on our inner world our outer world will alchemise. When your body is in alignment with your life purpose your purpose lines up with your life. We become conscious leaders in our families, in our neighbourhood, our community, in our circle of influence.

Marianne Williamson once wrote, "I will go at the slowest part of me." That's what conscious StressLess leaders do.

Their lives are integrated with habits, rituals, and beliefs, which minimise the stress in their lives, which in turn keeps them in the groove of life.

Robin Sharma, author of The Monk who Sold his Ferrari, says that we should lead without title. I totally dig that. Even if we are the cleaner in a shopping centre or the checkout chick at Woolworths, we should all do what we do with pride, excellence, and gratitude.

This standard alone will alleviate so much stress in your life. Even if you hate your job, or if you long for something different, do what you do now with excellence and use it as a steppingstone on your extraordinary path to fulfilment.

Conscious communication with your inner self will set you apart from everyone else for life. Being aware of your beliefs, your internal dialogue, your thoughts and feelings, and the physical sensations in your body can literally heal your life.

Our truth leads us to our divine potential. When we really, truly love ourselves and honour the truth of who we are, we break through whatever limits us. Creativity explodes, serendipity dances with synchronicity, and life as we know it will never be the same again.

The Pace of Grace leads us to our divine potential; it is how we access all that God has planned for us. It is a choice we make each and every day to love ourselves. To forgive ourselves and to want what is ours to have.

When we adopt a StressLess lifestyle we become what I term fully awake and fully at rest. Fully awake means to be completely present and conscious, grounded in the NOW moment, vibrant, alert and actively allowing the fullness of your intuition to come through you.

Fully at rest means to be operating from your para-sympathetic nervous system where you are in rest-and-relax state. This is where your whole body is at a gentle peace and harmony.

When we operate from this place, grace has free reign to take control and guide us into our divine potential, free from the constrictions with which we put on ourselves.

Both of these states are possible at the same time, and we can learn to instantly turn them on once we have cleared the blockages which prevent us accessing them.

Our body aligns with its natural state, free of toxicity, blocks from chronic stress, dis-ease, and stress, then the organs and systems have a chance to completely recharge when resting.

Then when you go about your day, your body can operate at optimal capacity, being fully awake, present, and charged with a magnified life force, where all areas of life start to come into balance.

For example, if you are experiencing awesome relationships but your finances are in the gutter, when your body is fully rested and fully awake, life has a chance to work for you. It can start to bring in new opportunities so that your bank balance can grow. Or it will provide you with challenges so that you can learn the lessons you need to learn in order to stop self-sabotaging your finances.

We all want the same things: to love and be loved, to matter, to feel worthy, and to be the best we can be, yet we let our thoughts get in the way of experiencing all of this. We rush around trying to prove ourselves, and all we gain in the process is to feel like we are still not good enough. We race after this goal and that goal, all the time forgetting that the ultimate goal is to know peace, joy, and love.

We live unconscious lives, moving with whatever pace society dictates, but life has a different pace, and it's here where you step off the treadmill and onto a road that will lead you towards more happiness than you can imagine. This road is not governed by dictatorship; it is not fuelled with unkindness and fear. This road is your road; you decide where it leads, you dictate the outcome, and you determine the elements it is made up of. You get to decide how fast or how slow you go based on divine guidance.

This road can be made up of untruths and fears, it can be ruled by the ego, and based on the premise that this is the way it's always been done. Or it can be the road less travelled, the one where truth lights your way, where there is only love, and where choices made from grace and mercy result in a kinder world for all species.

It's your choice: are you going to let stress, struggle, and fatigue keep you on the treadmill, always seeing the same things, never getting anywhere, just repeating the same day every day? Or are you going to choose ease, joy, and abundance, living life at the Pace of Grace and creating a StressLess Revolution?

I pray you come and evolve with me xx

Acknowledgements

Firstly I would like to acknowledge the fact that this book was born from what I perceived as a setback, which resulted in unapologetic self-love for myself, a deep connection for our animal species, and a grand vision for humanity.

I love how life can take our deepest mess and alchemise it into our greatest message. Each day as I sat down to write, I prayed that this process be one full of ease and flow. The Pace of grace was a joy to create as it came to me and through me each and every day.

I would like to thank my amazing husband who supported me in having the time and freedom to focus only on my writing. Your friendship and love are my dearest joys in life, and I count my blessings each and every day that I get to do life with you.

Diggity and Delhi, my beautiful fur babies: you are both gifts and you bring so much energy and fun into our lives. I feel so lucky that I get to be your mama.

To all the people in this book who make an appearance through my stories. Your contribution is what has shaped my life to what it is today; I wouldn't have it any other way.

To my amazing editor Anita: your skills and comments were a godsend, thank you, thank you, thank you.

And to enRich Retreat & Spa: what a beautiful part of the world to end up taking a sabbatical into wellness. Thank you for being my safe haven and my soft place to fall. Whilst you may no longer be a physical destination, the energy and intention behind your creation still lives on in cyber space in the form of an online program called RetreatMe.

RetreatMe is the perfect companion for this book and provides hand holding and support if you are serious about changing your life and effortlessly adapting to the energy of this new world.

You can find out more at https://www.karinastephens.com/retreat-me/

ABOUT THE AUTHOR

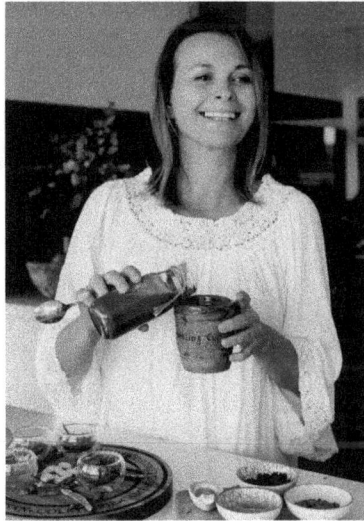

Karina Joy Stephens is an award-winning entrepreneur, author, Energy Guide, and animal advocate.

She has spent over thirty years in the health and wellness industry, initially training as a nurse, and then going on to be a personal trainer and holistic massage therapist. She is a qualified Wellness Coach, trained in Louise Hay 'Heal your Life' program and Rachael Jayne Groover's, The Art of Feminine Presence body of work, and completed the Raw Food Nutrition course from David Wolfe and the Body Mind Institute.

Together with her husband, Ian Stephens, she operates Enrich Training & Development, an international training and development company specialising in transformational change.

Inspired to create a sanctuary for people to retreat and renew, Karina founded the enRich Retreat & Spa in 2012 and won an international "Best Australasian Day-Spa Award". What was next was adrenal fatigue and exhaustion. Having experienced first-hand how stress affects us on a physical, energetic, emotional, and spiritual level, she became the CEO of her own wellness. Through her own research and experimentation, Karina found a different pace to life, one she has come to term "The Pace of Grace".

As an entrepreneur, writer, speaker, and wellness coach she promotes revolution through evolution, becoming the best version of ourselves possible so that we can create a kinder, gentler world.

She is also thrilled to bring enRich Retreat & Spa, her award-winning spa, into the online world with https://www.karinastephens.com/retreat-me/ creating a space for people to attend virtual retreats, workshops, and classes, all in the comfort of their own home and in their own time, without the huge expense.

When she is not travelling the world you will find her at home on the beautiful Sunshine Coast of Australia, dancing with her dogs and chillin' with her man.

What's your energetic signature?

Change your energetic signature,
transform your life?

Interested?

Take the free masterclass and learn how to analyse your energetic
signature and then learn how to change it in order to transform any
area of your life.

Visit the link for more info

https://www.karinastephens.com/ayes-landing/

www.ingramcontent.com/pod-product-compliance
Lightning Source LLC
Chambersburg PA
CBHW052134270326
41930CB00012B/2880